ABC'S of Alzheimer's Disease

◆

A Shared Reality by Me and My Shadow

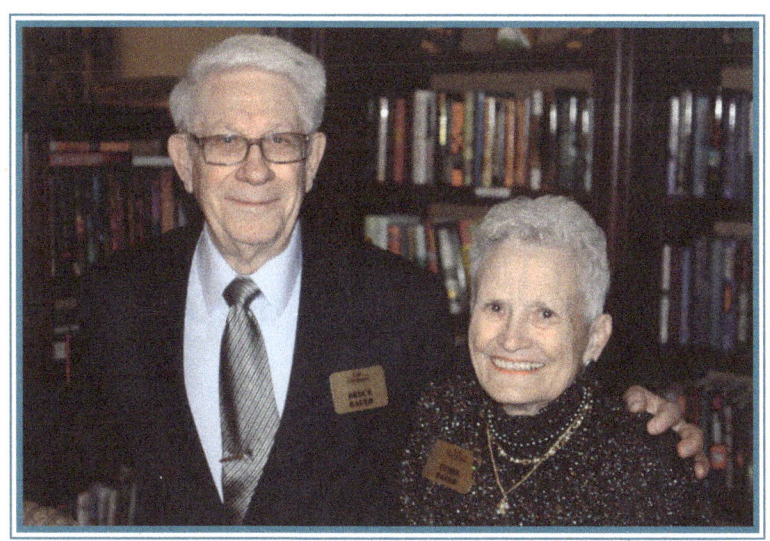

BRUCE BAUER

ISBN 978-1-64300-948-3 (Paperback)
ISBN 978-1-64559-283-9 (Hardcover)
ISBN 978-1-64300-949-0 (Digital)

Copyright © 2019 Bruce Bauer
All rights reserved
First Edition

All rights reserved. No part of this publication may be reproduced, distributed, or transmitted in any form or by any means, including photocopying, recording, or other electronic or mechanical methods without the prior written permission of the publisher. For permission requests, solicit the publisher via the address below.

Covenant Books, Inc.
11661 Hwy 707
Murrells Inlet, SC 29576
www.covenantbooks.com

Dedication and Acknowledgments

This book is dedicated to my wife of fifty-seven years who has been my inspiration and partner throughout our marriage. She was not only one of the first female scientists for NASA, but is also an inspirational mother for her children. Thank you, Ethel, the love of my life.

I would like to acknowledge the editorial help that I received from the late Marilyn LaRocque and Jennifer Zobelein, along with the proof reading provided by Dr. William Stephan the counsel and guidance throughout our journey by our neurologist Dr. Charles Bernick, and encouragement provided by Dr. Robert White.

Contents

Preface 7
Introduction 9

Section 1   Alzheimer's Disease—the Patient 11

1   Pride, Enjoyment, and Pain 13
2   Learning 32
3   Caregiving 56

Section 2   Alzheimer's Disease—Research 91

4   Clinical Trials 93
5   The Brain 123
6   Alzheimer's Disease (AD) Research 154
7   The Future 188
8   Understanding Alzheimer's Disease 220
References 249

Section 3   Appendix 259

Appendix A: Definitions 261
Appendix B: Websites 273
Appendix C: Alzheimer's Disease (AD) Timeline 275
Appendix D: AN-1792 Case Study 279
Appendix E: PET Scan Tracers 295

Preface

What is the status and reality of Alzheimer's disease (AD) at the end of 2018? Most current publications appear to have been issued five to twenty years ago. In general, these publications are either a caregiver's story, a neurologist's story, or medical academia experiences. At the time of issue, these publications provided useful information. Some include medical explanations of the brain and AD.

ABCs of Alzheimer's Disease: a Shared Reality by Me and My Shadow provides a 2018 research and evidence-based reality of not only Alzheimer's disease research, but also an ongoing seventeen-year patient-caregiver journey with behavioral stage decline guidance, using the Mini Mental State Exam (MMSE) along with clinical trial protocol explanation and trial experience including a Significant Adverse Events (SAE).

The book brings an up-to-date view of AD and genetic research that includes the latest technology contributions, discoveries, governance issues, research challenges, obstacles, probabilities, uncertainties, and realism. In addition, not only does the book address the paradigm shift to preclinical/presynaptic issues, it also offers outside-the-box ideas and suggestions such as elimination of clinical trial placebo cohort groups and low income/diversity solutions.

ABCs of Alzheimer's Disease is a story of Bruce and Ethel's journey along with a historical journey of AD from autopsy to PET scan research, including technology and genetic discoveries as well as providing potential for the education and/or training of patients, caregivers, primary care doctors, nurses, physician assistants, license nurse practitioners, certified nurse assistant, institutional care personnel, in-home health personnel, hospital personnel, educators, and politicians facing the future AD tsunami. In addition, this book can be a supplement document for geriatric schooling as well as enlightening and educating our political leaders (all three branches of government) and their staffs.

Introduction

Termed the health "tsunami" of the senior population, Alzheimer's disease (AD) connotes a slide into memory loss, which, over time, erases names and faces of family and friends. Normal functioning becomes impossible. The cause is unknown and there is no known cure. Through genetics, high risk factor genes, and DNA mutations are identified. Research provides hope. As life nears its end, love and care are needed.

Bruce and Ethel Bauer have been married for fifty-six years. They each have taken more than thirty years of engineering experience with General Electric and NASA into a retirement. Included was the challenge of AD for Ethel, whose beautiful brain once developed the slingshot trajectory used on Apollo 13. Now, they have been coping with her Alzheimer's for over sixteen years.

Before this writing, Bruce discussed with Ethel whether she was comfortable sharing their experiences.

She asked, "Why do we need to do this? We are happy. I'm still alive and doing okay."

Bruce said, "Maybe it would help others know they can be happy like you."

Ethel agreed.

Cheerful, attractive, fit, and energetic, Ethel, seventy-seven, seems in tune with life. Only when conversation swirls around her do you suspect something may be amiss. One evening, when Ethel saw an *exit* sign, she fixated on it, asking repeatedly, "What is that? What is that?" An answer did not sink in. Only after she and a friend walked to the *exit* sign and when the door, sign, and their relationships were explained did she drop the subject, seemingly satisfied. Thereafter, Bruce made sure there was nothing disruptive in her line of sight. Bruce is her guardian angel. That episode was four years ago. Now, as Ethel continues past her eightieth year, she has been over two years in the Ronald Reagan Memory Support Suites at Las Ventanas Retirement Community in Las Vegas, NV.

Bruce decided sixteen years ago to learn about the disease. He followed research by using the internet, read many books, submitted recommendations to the National Plan to Address AD, and self-educated himself on the brain through lessons from The Great Courses: *Understanding the Brain, Understanding Genetics,* and *Understanding the Human Body*. Bruce has written over fifty articles about AD and the brain, which he has shared with residents in Las Ventanas Continuing Care Community in Las Vegas, and, with many friends. These articles have become the background for his book.

ABCs of Alzheimer's Disease has three objectives as well as being both narrative and explanatory. The first three chapters contain the first objective, a narrative description of Ethel and Bruce's life journey and their experiences with AD. The second objective is met by the remaining chapters, which explain the technical complexity of AD medical research as well as its impact relative to the brain. This information allows primary care doctors, nurses, institutional and family caregivers, or an average college graduate (if they are motivated) to attain an understanding of AD. These chapters also provide a mini-historic insight into AD through referenced research evidence along with windows of understanding into clinical trials, the three levels of research, realistic expectations of the disease, and Bruce's basic description of the brain relative to AD. The appendixes that provide background information and tools for increased learning such as medical definitions, websites, etc. meet the third objective.

ABCs of Alzheimer's Disease imparts a foundation for understanding AD and provides reference tools to those motivated to expand their knowledge of the disease.

SECTION 1

Alzheimer's Disease— the Patient

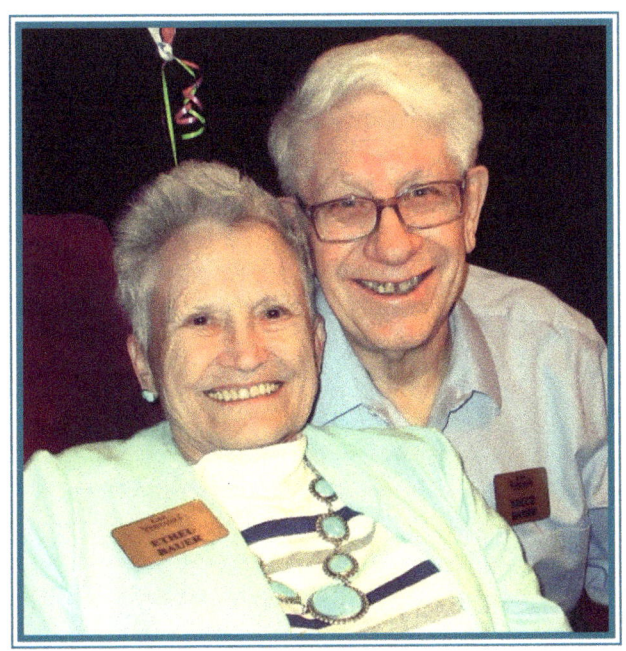

Patient – Caregiver

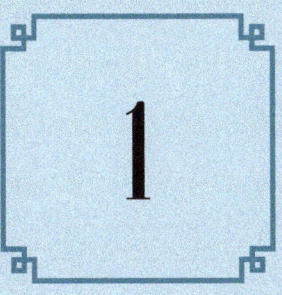

Pride, Enjoyment, and Pain

Alzheimer's disease (AD) is one of the greatest medical challenges of the twenty-first century. This is because of the increase in human lifespan brought about by the advancements made in technology, science, and education during the twentieth century. The latter part of that century saw a significant increase in senior aging. Lifespans of seniors reached into nine decades, and there were many centenarians. Along with a longer lifespan came a greater potential for Alzheimer's symptoms to appear. As the symptoms became more fully diagnosed, public awareness increased. Fortunately, medical knowledge increased immensely with technology benefits from the Apollo space program and the introduction of the microchip. The microchip led to a massive improvement in computers, the atomic force microscope, magnetic resonance imaging (MRI), and the internet. Medical science improved with donations of brains from those who died with AD. Medical universities established laboratories for dementia research along with working alongside the pharmaceutical industry on clinical trials. However, the complexity of the brain has thus far presented unsolvable problems. Patients were encouraged to make lifestyle changes such as diet and exercise to delay AD. Caregivers, with little or no knowledge of the disease, also had problems with understanding AD. For anyone motivated to learn about AD, this book should help.

Dr. Shin's Diagnosis

Returning to Las Vegas from a five-week trip to Europe, Bruce and Ethel had an appointment with Dr. Shin (primary care) on October 11, 2001. The doctor was completing Ethel's yearly physical with a series of questions. He gave us a diagnosis for Ethel that not only changed our lives, but also sent Bruce pursuing education again. Dr. Shin said Ethel had Alzheimer's disease and arranged for a neurological confirmation by Dr. Diaz, who ordered blood tests to determine if Ethel carried the ApoE4 gene allele that indicated a high risk for AD. She had it. Ethel's father and grandfather had both died of the disease, and the ApoE4 gene allele had passed to her. Dr. Shin's diagnosis was correct. Dr. Charles Bernick's neurological opinion was confirmation. Dr. Bernick became our permanent neurologist. He later helped open the Keep Memory Alive Brain Center in Las Vegas that later merged with the Cleveland Clinic. Dr. Bernick measured Ethel's score from the Mini-Mental State Examination (MMSE) at thirty, the highest score, but indicated that Ethel probably had mild cognitive impairment (MCI). However, due to her high intelligence, it would probably be a long time before any significant symptoms of Alzheimer's would appear. He was right. Since time was on our side, we decided to continue life as we always had while Bruce searched for knowledge, following his motto: *"Seek not the trust of medical doctors for your health issues; seek the knowledge to intelligently discuss your health issues with medical doctors."*

Therefore, in 2001, as a new caregiver, Bruce became acquainted with AD and set out to understand more about this terrible disease. In addition to learning about the complex brain, Bruce discovered he also needed to learn about other areas such as stages of AD, terminology, caregiving, nursing homes, biomarkers, researcher's tools, clinical trials, the national plan, lifestyle, and diet—all contributing to a caregiver's capability for *realistic* patient care. So, where do people turn to understand what to expect in the future?

The challenge for Bruce was to gain the knowledge needed to understand and discuss AD with Dr. Bernick and other medical professionals. Bruce's knowledge of AD was zero. He asked Dr. Bernick if Ethel had seven to ten years, to which Dr. Bernick replied *yes*. It was 2002, and with ten years of retirement behind them, Bruce and Ethel were thankful for their travels, where and when they went, and what they learned. The cruises, Tauck Tours, GE club tours, Elderhostel trips, and other trips Bruce planned all provided a variety of travel and education while increasing knowledge by seeing many wonderful countries, cultures, and economic situations that made them truly appreciate the United States.

This was not the time for self-pity. Instead, Bruce followed Doris Day's song "Que Sera, Sera" (Whatever will be, will be). The challenge and goal for the future was to understand and deal with a disease for which there was no known cause or cure and with medications of unknown benefit. Bruce was thankful for his engineering training and that he kept up with technology advances, which allowed him to use the internet. That became his school of the future.

Ethel Heinecke Bauer

On November 12, 1937, Ethel Heinecke was born in Troy, NY, to Dr. Howard Elwin and Grace Ethel Heinecke. Dr. Heinecke held doctorate degrees in both electrical engineering and physics from Rensselaer Polytechnic Institute in Troy, NY. He was a professor at the institute, teaching physics and electrical engineering. Grace received her RN degree from the University of Michigan. Though Ethel was Grace's first child, Ethel had an older half-sister, Joan Heinecke. Joan's mother had died in the childbirth of Joan, seven years earlier. Her paternal grandmother initially raised Joan.

World War II was looming, and the military needed scientific help in weapons development. Dr. Heinecke was not drafted because he was the sole supporter of his wife, his mother, his father (who had Alzheimer's disease), and two children, Joan and Ethel. Nevertheless, the government wanted his talents, and he became a civilian employee of the government in 1938.

The family moved to Montgomery, AL, where Dr. Heinecke began his lifelong career as a government scientist. When Ethel was two years old, her dad transferred to a secluded weapons testing area (now named Eglin Air Force Base) in the Florida panhandle near Ft. Walton Beach. He was instrumental in perfecting the Norden Bombsight during World War II and was involved in all the major bombing campaigns such as the Normandy invasion as well as the Trinity Test of the first atomic bomb.

Nineteen forty-six became a significant year for the Heinecke family. Grace delivered Ethel's brother (Howard C. Heinecke) in January, and later that year Dr. Heinecke was the recipient of the highest honor conferred to a civilian at that time, the Presidential Certificate. Dr. Heinecke joined a distinguished list of the country's outstanding aerial scientists, including such men as Igor Sikorsky (Sikorsky Helicopters), John Northrop (Northrop-Grumman), Glenn L Martin (Martin-Marietta), and Lawrence Bell (Bell Helicopters). Ethel inherited Dr. Heinecke's scientific mind and, unfortunately, Dr. Heinecke's gene allele (ApoE4)—believed to be a high-risk factor for AD—from which Dr. Heinecke died on August 15, 1991.

Ethel and her family lived in Valparaiso, FL, a small town jutting out into Choctawhatchee Bay. Swimming, water skiing, and fishing were her most popular sports. Ethel was quite a tomboy, playing softball, volleyball, shuffleboard, horseshoes, etc. She also excelled as a swimmer and caught fish with the best of them. She still recalls swimming and animatedly illustrates how she swam across the bay for a movie at the town of Niceville and tells people how she tied a helium balloon to her swimsuit so boaters would see her in the water.

Though her father stressed getting *A*s in school, his vision for his daughter's future was the stereotypical image of the time: a homemaker and mother. However, Ethel had her own dreams and determination to show her father that she had higher ambitions. While attending Choctawhatchee High School in Shalimar, FL, Ethel's high school selected her to be its representative at Florida's *Girl State* (a week of acting as a representative in State government) at the capital in Tallahassee, Fl.

After graduating with honors from Choctawhatchee High School in 1955, Ethel went to Montgomery, AL, for secretarial training and worked as a secretary for one year to earn tuition for entrance to Huntingdon College in Montgomery. She continued working while in college in such jobs as a professor's aide, tutor, college food server, and part-time accounting secretary. This was in addition to other summer jobs at Eglin Air Force Base as secretary, freight traffic clerk, and then two enjoyable summers as an engineering aide. She paid her own way through college with these jobs. In 1960, Ethel graduated with two degrees—a BS in mathematics and a BA in business administration.

During her college career, she served as a member of the honor board and was a class officer and president of the Athletic Association. Some of her honors included being among the top ten in her graduating class, receiving the *Wall Street Journal* Student Achievement Award, and a Ford Foundation scholarship to Vanderbilt University for pursuing a master's degree in mathematics.

Bruce Bauer

On April 13, 1933, in the German section of South St. Louis, MO, Bruce became the third son of Gregory George and Helen Mary (nee Schuhwerk) Bauer. Due to family hard times, neither Gregory nor Helen finished grade school. With German Catholic parents, nuns schooled Bruce in grade school and religious brothers in high school. This contributed beneficially to Bruce's value system. However, his scholastic education did not instill the fundamentals required in later life.

Bruce's childhood revolved around family, church, and friends. Economic conditions were bad, and hand-me-downs were the name of the game. Summers were hot, and there was no air conditioning. Bruce loved sports and played baseball and soccer. After high school in 1951, he went to work as a government employee classified as a cartographer, learning how to make maps.

In May 1953, Bruce received a letter from President Eisenhower that drafted him to serve his country as the Korean War was ongoing. Bruce reported in June 1953 to Camp Chaffee in Arkansas for basic training. After basic training, Bruce was ordered to Salzburg, Austria, instead of the Korean war zone. Because of his work as a cartographer, Bruce became part of the headquarter intelligence operation, working with a captain and sergeant, with responsibility to employ native Europeans to remap Austria. After duty in Salzburg, Bruce received an honorable discharge. The benefit of European travel and a military assignment with an intelligence operation that consisted of eighteen enlisted personnel and eighteen officers along with civilian personnel influenced Bruce's future.

In September 1955, stimulated during his military career by his officers and peers along with the GI Bill and summer work, Bruce took advantage of having a chance at a college education. His older brother Ray told him that the most important thing to take away from a college education was to learn how to think for yourself and how to find answers to issues you do not understand. Since the GI Bill covered only three and a half years, Bruce took twenty to twenty-three hours of engineering courses per semester to attain his bachelor of science in electrical engineering (BSEE) from the Missouri School of Mines and Metallurgy. While in college, Bruce joined Theta Kappa Phi Fraternity and served as treasurer and president.

Upon graduation in January 1959, Bruce travelled to Johnson City, New York, in February to start a lifelong career (thirty-three years) with the General Electric Company. In April 1960, GE sent Bruce to Eglin Air Force Base in Florida as part of a team conducting flight tests of a GE analog bombing computer in the F-105 aircraft.

One Sunday afternoon in June 1960, Charlie Frank (a Republic Aircraft crew chief) invited Bruce to go water skiing. Charlie introduced Bruce to Ethel Heinecke, and they spent a wonderful summer water skiing and fishing.

Ethel had accepted a Ford Foundation scholarship (full tuition and living expenses) and was leaving in September for Vanderbilt University in Nashville, TN. After one semester into the program and doing very well scholastically, Ethel decided to jump at the opportunity to join Dr. Werner von Braun's team with NASA in Huntsville, AL. Her fascination with rockets began.

Meanwhile, Bruce pursued Ethel with weekend long distance trips to Nashville, Tennessee, and Huntsville, Alabama. The long-distance romance paid off on September 23, 1961, as Ethel and Bruce were married. Ethel returned to work at Eglin. One of Ethel's responsibilities was developing flight paths and dispersion analyses for three-stage rockets shot into the upper atmosphere for various military applications. One classified mission was Firefly Ethel.

Bruce and Ethel

For the next eighteen months, Ethel and Bruce enjoyed the beautiful area of northwest Florida that later became known as the Miracle Strip. With sugar-like sand beaches stretching from Pensacola to Panama City, the Gulf of Mexico offered a lifestyle that is irreplaceable in today's overpopulated world. Sunday afternoons were spent water skiing with friends behind their boat on a calm bayou. The day ended with a beach cookout of T-bone steaks and baked potatoes on the grill. There were afternoons after work when they took fishing gear and their boat and went into the gulf to catch a King Mackerel for the evening meal. On overnight fishing trips out of Panama City that went far out into the gulf, they would catch grouper, amberjack, scamp, and red snapper. This was a wonderful life.

Bruce's job at Eglin was complete in 1963, and he transferred with GE to Huntsville, AL. Ethel returned to NASA at Marshall Spaceflight Center. Both Ethel and Bruce were deeply involved with all the Apollo flights to the moon and back and later with the NASA Skylab Projects. GE contracted with NASA to check out Apollo's Saturn I and Saturn V launch vehicles. Bruce was an engineer assigned to the instrument unit checkout equipment that controlled the stages of the launch vehicle. After receiving an award given to one person in a thousand, Bruce received a promotion, becoming the instrument unit manager.

While working at NASA George C. Marshall Space Flight Center's Aero Astrodynamics Laboratory, Ethel developed the flight trajectories for going to the moon and back for all the Apollo flights. What is aero astrodynamics?

Aero astrodynamics is the practical application of flight mechanics, astroballistics, propulsion theory, and allied fields to the problem of planning and directing the trajectories of space vehicles.

Ethel's was one of NASA's Marshal Space Flight Center women scientists. Pictured in the Figure 1.1, she is front and center in an Aero Astrodynamics Laboratory 1967 group picture. She stood out in the group of male engineers and scientists who accepted and respected her.

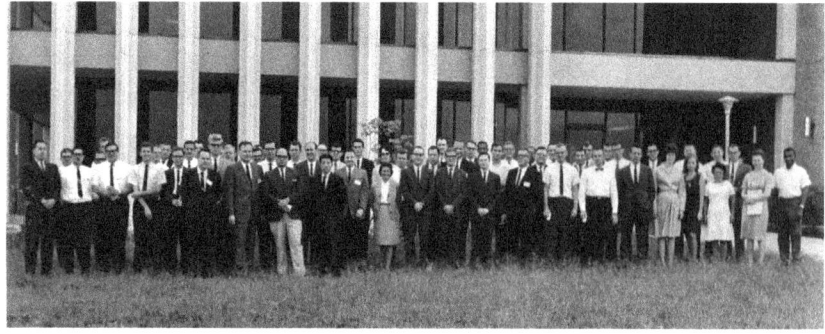

Figure 1.1. 1967 Aero Astrodynamics Laboratory Personnel.

On June 21, 1971, Dr. Eberhard Rees honored Ethel with a certificate, showing her Marshall Space Flight Center's nomination for the 1971 Federal Woman's Award (Figure 1.2). The nomination's summary read: "Mrs. Ethel H. Bauer is being nominated for the Federal Woman's Award for her outstanding contribution to the development and implementation of techniques which are directly applicable to Earth Resources and Earth Surveys Analysis utilizing the Skylab-A Space Mission. These contributions involved supervision of and direct participation in the procedures necessary to make the analysis meaningful.

Because of the complexity of the nature of the problem, it was necessary for a great deal of individual effort, especially during the terminal phase of the project, when everyone wanted answers "yesterday." The handling by Mrs. Bauer of this delicate phase speaks well for her ability and dedication.

The nomination's supporting documentation included the following:

1. "She helped pave the way for the first lunar orbit by the Apollo 8 crew, the subsequent landing on the moon, the 'free return' gravity swing past the moon used by the Apollo 13 crew, following a problem with the spacecraft.
2. She contributed to developing targeting procedures for U.S. manned lunar missions, which started in 1968.
3. She outlined procedures for guiding the rocket's third stage, which propels astronauts from earth orbit to a target just ahead of the moon.
4. She participated in developing the 'sling shot' method of disposing of the spent rocket stage, after it thrusts the Apollo crews to the moon.
5. She modified the trajectory of later missions to cause the spent third stage to impact on the moon for an added experiment bonus."

The free-return trajectory commonly called a slingshot, was available for all flights to the moon and back, *not* landing on the moon. It was the reference trajectory for a safe return to earth if anything went wrong on the way to the moon. When Apollo 13 needed it, it worked.

While in Huntsville, Ethel gave birth to Greg, Bill, and Ann. Bill died in 1968 at an early age of three from severe problems during birth. Ethel, at the forefront of

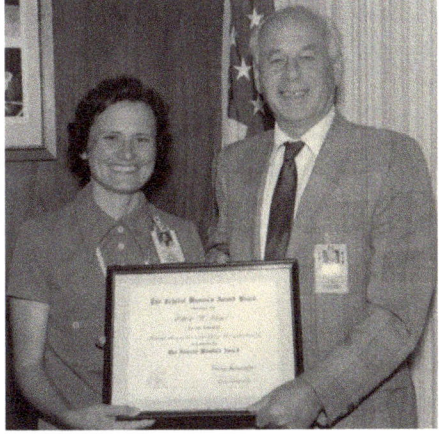

Figure 1.2. Federal Woman's Award Nomination.

women in science, was listed in the 1965 edition of Outstanding Young Women in America, but she was prouder of the recognition shown by her father. Bruce's view of her outstanding achievement was as a wife and working mother in the era when the scientific community first began accepting women.

Ethel's most outstanding quality was her personality and continually positive and happy outlook with everyone she met. While in Huntsville, Ethel loved to play poker with a group of women. The phone would ring almost every evening to see if she was available for the floating poker game. Another interest was card and magic tricks that she perfected to the delight and wonderment of her friends.

When the Apollo program ended, new opportunities resulted in the next phase of life and work in Saratoga, CA. GE transferred Bruce to work on nuclear energy. Ethel transferred with NASA to Ames Research Center, where she was initially involved in technology transfer of satellite data for management of crops and control of ragweed for the five Western states. This provided Ethel the opportunity to know scientists from Washington, Oregon, Idaho, Montana, and California, whom she organized not only into a working group but enticed to enjoy her home cooking and an evening poker game. The following memos that she received when she retired best show Ethel's outstanding contribution to NASA at both Marshall Space Flight Center and Ames Research Center. The first note is from her immediate boss, John Givens. The next is an eloquent letter from the director of Ames Research Center that captured Ethel and her career. The last letter is from NASA Headquarters in Washington DC.

ABC'S OF ALZHEIMER'S DISEASE

January 30, 1993

Ethel:

I have just taken that step of removing "Bauer" from the QuickMail list and I must say it was not an easy task, bringing more than one tear to my eyes. I know your efforts on behalf of NASA, Ames and the Centrifuge Facility Project have made major contributions to the successes of these organizations throughout your career. But I guess what makes me so emotional about seeing you go is the contributions you have made to all of us personally and I think to a large extent to my growth as a manager over the years you have been here. So it was with heavy heart that I watched you leave yesterday. Let me thank you for your help, support and comfort when we were dealing with the difficult issues; technical, programmatic, or personnel. You will go down in my book as one of the outstanding people I have worked with over the years.

On a bright side, let me wish you and Bruce the best on your collective retirements. I am sure you folks will have a good time and know you will continue to give the same support to the people you come in contact in your retired life as you did to us around here. Let us know about your adventures in the Amazon or other interesting places you explore. We will make some effort at keeping you informed of all of the machinations of the NASA store as it wends its way through its bureaucratic life.

John G.

BRUCE BAUER

National Aeronautics and
Space Administration

Ames Research Center
Moffett Field, California 94035-1000

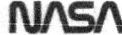

Reply to Attn of: SC:244-19/3-004

January 31, 1993

Ms. Ethel H. Bauer
Mail Stop 244-19
NASA-Ames Research Center
Moffett Field, CA 94035-1000

Dear Ethel:

May I add my best wishes to the many other wishes I'm sure you are receiving as you retire from employment with the Federal Government.

You have every right to feel very satisfied with the contributions you have made to Ames Research Center, and the National Aeronautics and Space Administration. Your total 32 years of Federal Government employment is an enviable record of accomplishment and service.

Your work on the Apollo Program at Marshall Space Flight Center and your work here at Ames in the Mission Analysis Division, the Earth Resources Observation programs, development of ground communications, and the Centrifuge Facility Project have always been of the highest quality. You have demonstrated outstanding dedication to getting the job done. You have served as a role model for young women engineers as one of NASA's first women in both engineering and management positions. In addition, your perceptive and caring approach to people has made significant contributions to getting the NASA mission accomplished and provided valuable personal support to those with whom you have worked. We thank you not only for your direct and significant contributions to the Ames mission, but also for the very large indirect contribution you have made by working with, mentoring, encouraging, guiding and supporting so many co-workers and subordinates. Your personal interactions have been an important part of your contributions.

We hope you will keep in touch with your many friends at Ames; you will certainly be missed in the day-to-day activities of the Center.

Again, best wishes for your new career as a retiree!

Sincerely,

Dale L. Compton
Director

Telephone: (415) 604-5000   FTS 464-5000   Central FAX: (415) 604-4003

ABC'S OF ALZHEIMER'S DISEASE

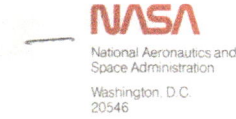

National Aeronautics and
Space Administration

Washington, D.C.
20546

Reply to Attn of: SBF   JAN 2 5 1993

Mrs. Ethel Bauer
Chief, Project Engineering Division
Centrifuge Facility Project Office
Ames Research Center
Moffett Field, CA 94035

Dear Ethel:

I would like to take this opportunity to express not only for myself but for the NASA Headquarters staff and the LESC and CSAT Support Contractor staffs, who had the pleasure to work with you over the years, our sincere thanks and appreciation to you for your outstanding performance in directing and overseeing the project engineering activity for the Centrifuge Facility project. Your leadership and ability to deal with a whole host of organizations, some of which you may want to forget, to further the goals of the CF project proved to be invaluable to the success of this program. It has not been easy to focus on our goal when it seems like program redirection will never end. But as we work through each set of problems our goal of achieving success becomes ever brighter. For the folks here in Washington, we will surely miss you and your support for achieving this goal.

The kind of dedication and enthusiasm you have displayed is exactly what is needed to make this program a success. We all will surely miss you and wish you the best in your retirement. But please remember Ethel, you should be very proud of your contributions to this program. They will not be forgotten.

Again, let me say thanks to you for a job well done.

Sincerely,

Lawrence P. Chambers
Lawrence P. Chambers
Manager, Life Sciences Space Station Freedom Program

A thank you note (below) internationally recognized Ethel's contribution, received from those she supported from Pietermaritzburg, South Africa.

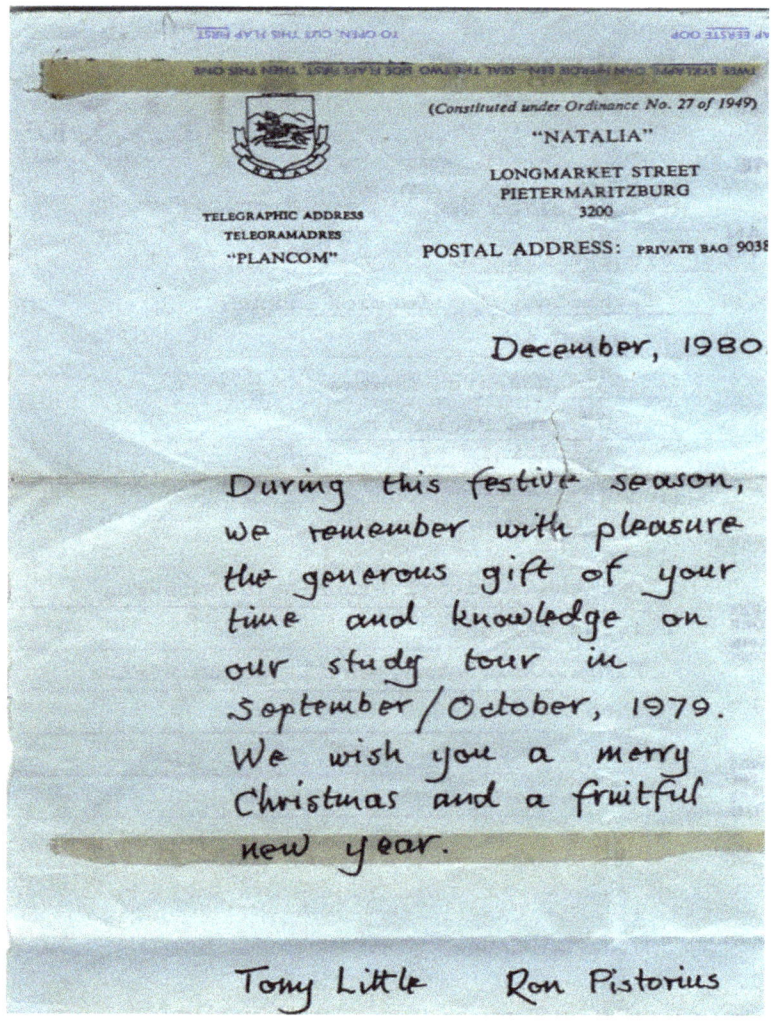

These years in Saratoga saw Greg and Ann grow from children into adulthood with the trials that all parents experience. Despite both working in challenging careers, Bruce and Ethel dedicated every hour off work to Greg and Ann. When not interfered by Greg or Ann's soccer, which Bruce coached, many weekends and holidays were spent skiing at Lake Tahoe during the winter months. Summertime often found them at their beach house in Santa Cruz, eating fresh salmon.

For thirty years spanning work and retirement, the family spent the last weekend in September, enjoying an abalone feast at a ranch about a hundred miles north of San Francisco. It began with coworkers diving for abalone and ended with Greg, Ann, and Alex (Ann's husband) and their friends diving and providing the abalone.

Christmas of 1981 found the family on a Western Caribbean cruise. Bruce retired from his engineering management position with General Electric in December 1992 at the age of fifty-nine after thirty-three years. Despite the offer of a promotion, Ethel retired in January 31, 1993, at the age of fifty-five after a thirty-two-year NASA career.

Our Retirement and Travel

Not satisfied with just two hours a day of exercise activities, Bruce decided not only to continue to take advantage of the GE travel club, but also to plan trips and explore what this educational travel for seniors called Elderhostel was all about. Returning from an Elderhostel trip to Zion National Park in October 1994, we took advantage of an invitation to spend a weekend as guests of Sun City Summerlin in Las Vegas, NV. There, we toured model homes and played golf. Upon returning home to Saratoga, a note was in the mailbox, saying someone was interested in buying our home. With Ethel's persistence to contact the people, we negotiated the sale of our house over the next few months. It happened so fast that we had to rent the house back until the end of March 1995. During that time, we travelled to Las Vegas to purchase a new home in Sun City Summerlin, a Del Webb retirement community.

On April 1, 1995, we moved from Saratoga, CA, to a rental home in the Sun City Retirement Community while our new home was completed. Our vision of active living became a reality as our hobby list started with taking up golf. Bruce added other interests: lapidary, silversmith, stained glass, genealogy, financial advisor, and finally becoming educated about Alzheimer's disease and writing. Meanwhile, Ethel became Nevada's Senior Women Table Tennis champion and participated in the Senior Olympics in Clearwater, Florida. She also had a Hole in One playing golf, participated in the sewing club, and became their block's party hostess and self-appointed welcoming person for new residents.

Traveling started before retirement with our first trip in 1990 to Germany, Austria, Slovakia, Hungary, and France. Highlights were the *Passion Play* in Oberammergau, a cruise on the Danube from Vienna to Budapest and back, and German Reunification day in Munich. A fourteen-day Mediterranean cruise with GE's travel group in 1992 concluded our preretirement travel.

After retirement, a fourteen-day GE Club cruise left Miami, the highlights being Barbados, Devil's Island in French Guiana, crossing the equator and heading to Brazil for a one-thousand-mile trip up the Amazon River to Manaus and a journey into the rain forest.

GE travel club then planned a fantastic seven-day September 1993 trip where we flew in a small Cessna to a Dude Ranch somewhere in Utah that included sleeping in a Calistoga Wagon. The next morning, we flew in a helicopter down to the Colorado River for three days and two nights of rafting through the Grand Canyon, sleeping along the banks under the stars. We ended our trip at the Hotel Mirage in Las Vegas for two days.

Our daughter Ann became Mrs. Ann Ross on April 23, 1994. After the wedding, Ethel and Bruce, along with Ethel's sister Joan and her husband John, departed for a four-week trip planned by Bruce to Scotland and England. We spent a week on the shore of Scotland's Lock Oich in a two-bedroom condo. From there it was a week in a three-bedroom home on the shore of Tourqey, a resort area on the English Channel. Two weeks in a two-bedroom penthouse apartment in the Soho district of London that was two blocks from the British Museum concluded the trip.

Bruce's highlights were the British Museum and Blenheim Palace (Winston Churchill's birthplace) that was a gift from Queen

Ann to John Churchill when she elevated him from Earl to the first Duke of Marlborough for his victory over France at Blenheim in 1703. Ethel's highlight was the Dungeons at The Tower of London.

Shortly after a September 1995 move into our new home, we joined the GE travel club's outstanding tour of South America. It started with a flight to Santiago, Chile for a few days, followed by a flight over the snowcapped Andes to Porta Arenas, and a two-day stay in Patagonia (Chile's National Park). This was followed by a flight to La Paz, Bolivia, landing at 14,000 feet and then to Lake Titicaca at 12,000 feet, where Bruce experienced altitude sickness. The final part of the trip included stops at the magnificent Cataratas Falls and then on to Buenos Aries. Bruce's highlights were many, including collecting Chilean lapis lazuli and Argentinian rhodochrosite for his lapidary hobby and seeing Patagonia and the Cataratas Falls. Ethel's highlights were the strenuous hiking in Patagonia and the view over the snowcapped Andes.

In May 1997, following Greg and Molly's April Wedding, we joined another unique GE Club tour—this time, Russia. This was just after Russia opened its country for American tours. We experienced the combination of the old Soviet Union and Russian attempts at capitalism. We landed at St. Petersburg and, as required, turned in our passports while staying at a very nice hotel. The hotel was gated and with armed guards. An overnight sleeper train took us from St. Petersburg to Moscow where we boarded a riverboat. After two days of Moscow touring, we proceeded down the Volga River to Kazan and back. Bruce's highlights of Russia were the Hermitage, Fabergé Eggs at the Kremlin, negotiating for Malachite at a Moscow flea market, and Catherine the Great's Palace. The poor economic conditions everywhere we went amazed Ethel.

In February 1998, we took a twenty-four-day Tauck Tour to Australia and New Zealand. Besides wonderful stays in Sidney and Melbourne, we spent two days in the Outback at Alice Springs with a sunset cocktail party at Ayers Rock. After a camel ride the next day, we proceeded to a swim at the Great Barrier Reef in Queensland. Then we traveled on to Auckland, New Zealand. Our visit to Christchurch included a helicopter flight to the top of Mt. Cook and a trip to

Milford Sound. Ethel's highlight was finding an opal necklace and earrings. Bruce's highlight was finding a four-volume set of books on Marlborough written by Winston Churchill (2,800 pages).

In July 1999, Bruce and Ethel took another unique GE Club tour of China. Highlights included Beijing's Tiananmen Square, the Great Wall of China, the Terracotta soldiers, a river trip down the Yangtze to Shanghai and a jade statue of Buddha.

In August 2001, Bruce, Ethel, her sister Joan and husband John took a four-week trip planned by Bruce to Switzerland, Austria, and Germany. We spent a wonderful summer week in the Interlaken area of Switzerland with a cog rail trip to the top of the Jungfrau and a tour through an ice cave. With short-sleeve weather, we watched hang gliders land in an open park while dining on the patio of an Interlaken café. After a boat trip across Lake Constance, we spent a week on the shore of Lake Constance at the Seehof Bed and Breakfast in the resort town of Meersburg, Germany. Through Bruce's genealogy work, we contacted a distant cousin on his maternal heritage side. Everyone enjoyed a wonderful evening of dining and talking, despite language difficulties.

A train ride took us next to Salzburg, Austria. (Bruce was stationed there in the service.) We were having dinner at a restaurant that Bruce frequented in 1954. As it happened, it was 9/11/2001, and the waiter took us into the kitchen where we saw on television the second airplane crash into the Twin Towers of the World Trade Center. With plans for Oktoberfest and connections with other cousins and ancestral birthplace visits, we arrived in Munich. The German people showed their grief for the victims of 9/11/2001 attack on the Twin Towers with an overwhelming array of flowers at Marianplatz. A real display of friendship by the German people was everywhere. Between Oktoberfest and an evening at the Hofbrau House, we experienced how the German people enjoy themselves. We took day trips to Regensburg, Augsburg, and Furth im Wald from where Bruce's paternal grandfather emigrated in 1890. Significant increased security was everywhere for our return trip to Las Vegas and the forthcoming news from Dr. Shin was a life-changing significant event—the Alzheimer's stage of life.

So, What Is Alzheimer's Disease?

Alzheimer's disease (AD) is a neurocognitive (brain) disorder under the umbrella of dementia. Simply stated, Alzheimer's disease (AD) is a loss of brain function that gradually gets worse over time. It affects memory, thinking, behavior, and, finally, body function. Dr. Aloysius Alzheimer discovered Alzheimer's disease in 1906.

In 1901, Dr. Alzheimer observed a patient named Auguste Deter at the Frankfurt Asylum. This fifty-one-year-old patient had strange behavioral symptoms, including a loss of short-term memory. In April 1906, Mrs. Deter died, and Dr. Alzheimer had the patient records and brain brought to Munich where he was working. Using the original microscope during an autopsy of Mrs. Dater's brain, he identified amyloid plaques and neurofibrillary tangles.

Dr. Aloysius "Alois" Alzheimer (14 June 1864–19 December 1915) was a Bavarian-born German psychiatrist and neurologist and a colleague of Emil Kraepelin. Dr. Alzheimer identified and published the first case of presenile dementia, which Kraepelin would later call Alzheimer's disease.

How to Learn About Alzheimer's Disease

With so many areas to explore, Bruce Bauer started with trying to establish a benchmark of where the research stood at the end of 2001. In hindsight, Bruce found no benchmarks. He found only very dedicated, highly intelligent researchers trying to unravel a very difficult problem while increasing their knowledge one failed trial at a time. After a 2002 internet search of the AN-1792 vaccine, which was in a phase two trial after promising phase one results for safety, Bruce was encouraged and motivated to continue his learning—which began a new career.

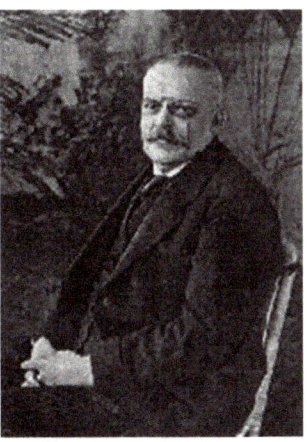

Figure 1.3. Dr. Alzheimer

Learning

Everyone knows that learning means going to school—maybe yes and maybe no. How many in the United States have gone to school but failed to learn? They may have learned other things (possibly inappropriate in some people's view). So, what is learning? At the beginning of life, it is the instinctive inputs from genes and parental care. From there, consider it as the sensory inputs (sight, hearing, touch, smell, taste) that the brain receives. These inputs are stored as memory and later become knowledge. Maturity brings values, events, and episodes, also stored in memory. These data provide the source for the executive function of the neocortex to create a higher order of intelligence. Current research evaluations have shown that clinical patients with higher levels of education tend to delay the decline process of Alzheimer's disease (AD) to which Ethel fits. So, where did this leave Bruce in his search to understand AD?

Many books, articles, media, conferences, and research publications attempt to describe a very complex AD. The communications in many of these publications have been technical and difficult for a nonprofessional to understand. Other books have chronicled decline paths from symptoms as viewed by caregivers. These sources contained valuable information and advice. Most specialized to a specific theme or storytelling as opposed to a comprehensive picture.

Bruce's learning started with pursuing AD knowledge. His challenge was simplification of the AD complexity, targeting a market for a book and learning the complexities in writing a book. Bruce learned AD complexities were so massive that simplification became a relative term. This influenced Bruce to target anyone with the desire and willpower to pursue knowledge. Bruce believes an AD tsunami will occur during the first half of the twenty-first century and will create the demand for knowledge by the baby boomer generation and beyond, along with primary care doctors, nurses as well as any people involved with geriatric care. The approaching AD tsunami is due to medical advances that have allowed people to live longer due to advances in medical treatment of physical organs but not the brain. As future demands for senior care overwhelm the medical profession and AD care providers, baby boomer caregivers will seek knowledge for managing care and expectations. Senior care is becoming a growth industry, demanding knowledgeable personnel at all levels of care. (Chapter 7, Outside the Box, suggests ideas for addressing this problem.) This book is intended to be a reference source for many of these people.

Bruce found that writing a book involved learning additional skills such as copyright research; computer word processing tools; graphics; referencing; editing; and rewrite, rewrite, rewrite. Existing source information guided Bruce, not only to learn about AD symptoms or tell stories or caregiving, but also to understand the brain, genetics, clinical trials, and research.

Bruce's learning approach was the following: (a) locate sources of information, (b) gain knowledge of AD, (c) learn about the brain and follow research, (d) learn to communicate with the reader and (e) share the benefits of learning, (f) identify "outside the box" ideas, (g) provide opinions from learning, (h) summarize, and (i) learn dementia.

Locate Sources and Information

Bruce began by attending Alzheimer's association meetings. The meetings provided another source of information with insight into the personal experiences of others. He observed caregivers' stress and the value of their venting. At the time, it was difficult to appreciate the caregiver's need to be able to talk with someone who could communicate back to him.

Books and the internet became the primary sources of learning in the early years. DVDs from The Great Courses along with the purchase of *Principles of Neural Science, Fifth Edition* also enhanced the learning process. E-mailed questions to researchers received responses that were amazing and gratifyingly appreciated.

Gain Knowledge of AD

The first step in learning is defining the problem. As indicated in chapter 1, Dr. Aloysius Alzheimer defined the problem in his first published report in which he called the disease senile dementia. Through an autopsy, he identified a sticky substance *as amyloid plaques and neurofibrillary tangles*. On twentieth century death certificates, senile dementia became an umbrella term that covered many brain disorders, of which AD was one. So, what are *amyloid plaques and neurofibrillary tangles*? Are there different types of AD? What are risk factors? What are the chances of inheriting the disease? What are the caregiver's issues and duties? What is a clinical trial? How does the brain work? What are symptoms? How does behavior change during the decline process? What are realistic future expectations? Why is AD so complex? These questions define the problem. Not only caregivers, but also researchers, primary care doctors, nurses, personal care aides, and government decision makers face these questions. Chapters 3 through 8 provide some answers, from which readers can learn and/or increase their knowledge of AD.

AD types in 2001 were early onset (EOAD), and late onset (LOAD), EOAD occurs before age sixty-five and as early as thirty.

Some EOAD patients inherit mutated genes of either presenilin 1 on chromosome 14 or presenilin 2 on chromosome 1. Familiar AD (EOFAD) classifies these patients. Non-FAD is sporadic AD or late onset (LOAD). LOAD, the more common form of the disease, occurs after age sixty-five. apolipoprotein E gene's allele E4 (ApoE4) is an inherited risk factor for LOAD. The link between genes and disease is not clear. Chapter 5, The Brain, will explain the evolution process. A blood test determined that *Ethel inherited the ApoE4 allele from her father.*

During the period between October 2001 (Ethel AD diagnosis) and this writing, Bruce has interacted with researchers via e-mail, clinicians via trials, our neurologist (Dr. Bernick), medical courses via The Great Courses, and books. These provided an appreciation of the struggles, frustrations, challenges, risks, and uncertainties accepted by the pharmaceutical companies, clinicians, researchers, politicians, and FDA decision makers. Bruce found medical terminology very difficult to understand. However, he searched the internet and read and reviewed many published papers. He began with a book (*AB Metabolism* by K. Takata et al).

Interaction with researchers by e-mail increased his respect and admiration of these professionals. Samples of the e-mail interactions that follow indicate the uncertainty at that time.

1. *July 27, 2004 e-mail to Anne Fagan*—Washington University, St. Louis, Mo. → Bruce's question was regarding a 2003 workshop identifying a clinical trial, Antecedent Biomarker in Alzheimer Disease 11/23/03, which stated, "Add younger cases to the clinical samples as antecedent AD changes may occur years or decades prior to the symptomatic expression of the disease," and whether Ethel could apply for this trial.

    August 5, 2004, e-mail from Anne Fagan (excerpts) → We know that the pathology of AD (e.g., amyloid plaques) starts some ten to twenty years before evidence of even the earliest clinical signs of the disease (e.g., memory problems). What this means in the real world is that there are millions of individuals, now in their forties and fifties, who have AD pathology starting in their brains but who don't even know it because they have no symptoms yet. Our goal is to be able to stop the disease from even starting. Being able to halt or even just slow its progression once it's already begun will do tremendous good! So, as you can see, Ethel is not a suitable candidate for our particular antecedent biomarker study, both because of her advanced age and the fact that she's already exhibiting some cognitive difficulties. If you have adult children who are between the ages of forty-five to sixty-four, these are the individuals we are recruiting for our study.

Bruce's Comment: It was 2014 (a decade later) before tools (PET scan tracer/radioactive isotopes) became available, and amyloid could be identified in the brain with certainty.

2. *March 3, 2005, e-mail to Dr. John Morris*—Washington University, St. Louis, Mo. Bruce's question → Is the brain/blood barrier well understood?

    March 4, 2005, e-mail from Dr. John Morris → The blood-brain barrier is not completely understood but much now is being learned. The brain contains blood (including the fluid component of blood—or plasma), but the blood is confined to the blood vessels of the brain.

3. *March 4, 2005, e-mail to Dr. David Holtzman*—Washington University, St. Louis, Mo. Bruce's question → Does the brain contain LDL cholesterol? I thought it only had HDL.

    March 6, 2005, e-mail from Dr. David Holtzman → The brain does not contain LDL. The brain produces a certain kind of HDL or high-density lipoprotein. The HDL in the brain are distinct from that in the plasma. The brain HDL are made in the brain and are not influenced by the diet, as far as we know. What influences brain HDL and what function it has is an active area of research but not yet understood.

4. *April 2006 Dr. Bernick's Invitation*—Bruce and Ethel's learning experience received a very pleasant surprise by an

invitation from Dr. Bernick of the Keep Memory Alive Foundation to attend the foundation's sponsored conference in Las Vegas, NV, titled Common *Threads Think Tank*. The conference had twenty distinguished researchers from foreign countries and the USA. There were participants from the pharmaceutical industry, research scientists, university professors, and various foundation science advisors. Dr. Bernick asked Ethel to share her experience from the Apollo program and her dealing with AD at this point. We stayed for only the morning session on the first day. For Bruce, the conference was like being in a foreign country where you did not know the language. It further emphasized the need to learn more about the disease. Listening to a discussion on mitochondria, led by M. Flint Beal from Weill Medical College at Cornell University, was stimulating—even though an unknown to Bruce. (Chapter 7 will provide more information about mitochondria.)

During a morning break, we talked with the late Dr. Leon J. Thal, chair of Department of Neuroscience, University of California, San Diego, and co-organizer of the conference. We also met Dr. Virginia Lee, director of the Center for Neurodegenerative Disease, University of Pennsylvania School of Medicine. Years later, Dr. Lee responded to an inquiry Bruce made regarding the tau protein and kindly provided her research paper on the subject.

After the break, Ethel addressed the researchers. She discussed her career at NASA. Ethel said that she suspected memory issues prior to retiring from her thirty-two-year career with NASA. Ethel encouraged them to meet a similar challenge that President Kennedy set for the Apollo program and find a cure for AD within the next ten years. They missed the deadline, but obstacles were not only far greater, there was also no political support. Looking back, we had so little knowledge and appreciation of the complexities researchers faced. The conference was a motivator for Bruce to continue his quest for AD knowledge.

Learn about the Brain and Follow Research

Bruce quickly found AD leadership was lacking in 2002. Academia was driving basic research, tools were evolving, pharmaceuticals were pursuing the next blockbuster drug, and everyone was learning. This shotgun pursuit was probably appropriate for the state of AD knowledge in the first decade of the twenty-first century. Later chapters will identify failed trials, genetic and technology breakthroughs, the brain, advocate success in achieving a national plan, and recognition of caregiver's issues. Bruce pursued knowledge based on the AD Model that he developed.

Bruce used the internet to pursue the state of research knowledge between 2003 and 2007, which led to many avenues of information from which he developed the AD Model (Figure 2.1). This model captured the issues occurring at the time. The AD Model, formulated into a six-section pie chart, identified major components of AD. Bruce chose current R&D, future R&D, tools, drugs & targets, diets, and vitamins as components of the model.

Current R&D was being driven by the amyloid cascade hypothesis (ACH) that suggested amyloid plaque caused neurofibrillary tangles. Therefore, focus was on beta and gamma secretase enzymes. A gamma secretase inhibitor targeted the amyloid precursor protein's (APP) beta amyloid peptide. Genetic research was identifying the genome. Computer and biomedical technology were developing support tools such as magnetic resonance imaging (MRI), large data analysis, genetic sequencing, brain banks, and radioactive isotopes for PET Scans. Based on his knowledge at the time, these issues seemed encouraging to Bruce (eternal hope).

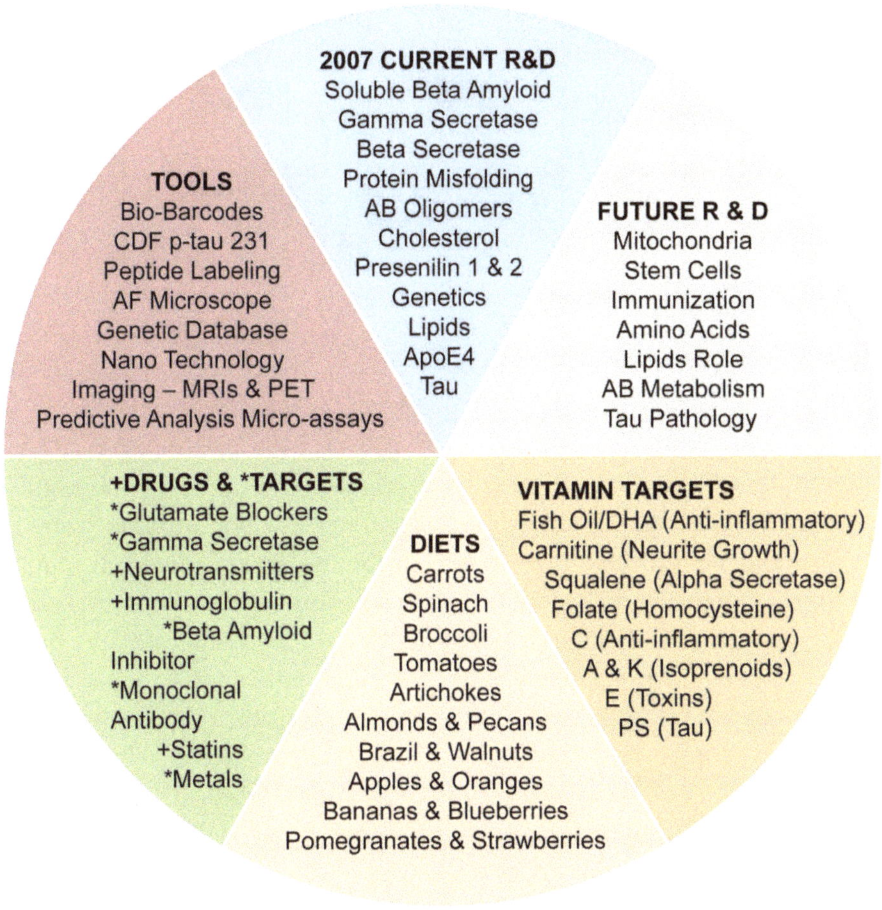

ABC'S OF ALZHEIMER'S DISEASE

2007 CURRENT R&D
Soluble Beta Amyloid
Gamma Secretase
Beta Secretase
Protein Misfolding
AB Oligomers
Cholesterol
Presenilin 1 & 2
Genetics
Lipids
ApoE4
Tau

TOOLS
Bio-Barcodes
CDF p-tau 231
Peptide Labeling
AF Microscope
Genetic Database
Nano Technology
Imaging – MRIs & PET
Predictive Analysis Micro-assays

FUTURE R & D
Mitochondria
Stem Cells
Immunization
Amino Acids
Lipids Role
AB Metabolism
Tau Pathology

+DRUGS & *TARGETS
*Glutamate Blockers
*Gamma Secretase
+Neurotransmitters
+Immunoglobulin
*Beta Amyloid
Inhibitor
*Monoclonal
Antibody
+Statins
*Metals

DIETS
Carrots
Spinach
Broccoli
Tomatoes
Artichokes
Almonds & Pecans
Brazil & Walnuts
Apples & Oranges
Bananas & Blueberries
Pomegranates & Strawberries

VITAMIN TARGETS
Fish Oil/DHA (Anti-inflammatory)
Carnitine (Neurite Growth)
Squalene (Alpha Secretase)
Folate (Homocysteine)
C (Anti-inflammatory)
A & K (Isoprenoids)
E (Toxins)
PS (Tau)

Figure 2.1. 2007 Alzheimer's Disease Guidance Model by Bruce

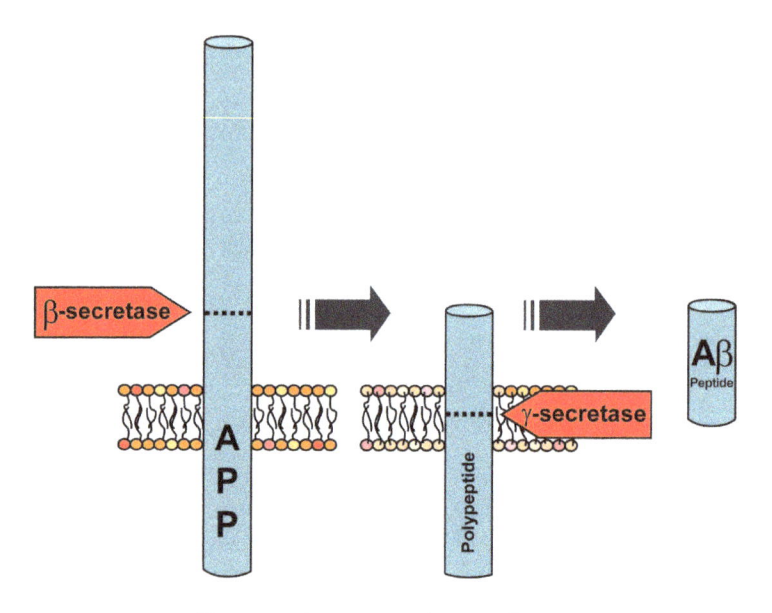

Fig. 2.2. APP to AB by I. Peltan.

The Alzheimer's Cascade Hypothesis (ACH) [Ref. 22 & 23] proposed that beta amyloid peptide AB$_{42}$ cascaded to cause neurofibrillary tangles* and neuron loss. (See chapter 6 for ACH additional information). Beta Amyloid is a peptide* formed from the amyloid precursor protein (APP) (Figure 2.2). The beta secretase enzyme cuts the APP protein forming a polypeptide* of ninety-nine amino acids. The gamma secretase enzyme then cuts the polypeptide. to form variable peptides consisting of either AB$_{40}$ or AB$_{42}$ amino acids. AB$_{40}$ is the soluble form. AB$_{42}$ aggregates to form a toxic plaque. An overproduction of APP occurs because of a mutation in the APP gene (*See Appendix A for definitions).

A protein's amino acids are defined by a gene's DNA. A gene has a one-to-one relationship with a protein, whereby it defines the protein's amino acid instruction set through DNA coding, thereby producing the protein to implement the instruction of the intended gene function.

Autopsies confirmed APP and tau proteins as suspects for late onset AD, in addition to the ApoE4 allele as a risk factor. An allele refers to a specific variation of a gene (one provided by the mother and one by the father). One of the proteins (amyloid precursor protein—APP) produces amyloid. The other protein (tau) normally acts like a set of railroad tracks for communications from inside the nucleus out to the external communication link. Chapter 6 addresses ACH and the two proteins.

By 2007, Bruce learned that the *future* offered many opportunities for career academics to pursue AD. So much was unknown. Bright spots were MRIs, genetics, technology advances, and radioactive tracers for PET Scans. Mitochondria, the brain's immune system, stem cells, DNA databases, and the tau protein were receiving attention. Chapters 7 and 8 address these.

Only acetylcholinesterase inhibitor drugs were available in 2002. These drugs were not obviously beneficial from a patient symptom point of view. This may be due to their target being too general as opposed to specific symptom-modifying targets. A new drug (Namenda) entered the marketplace in 2003.

Contrary to most organs in the human body, the brain has limitations for invasive techniques. Therefore, researchers were challenged to create innovative methods to pursue knowledge and understanding of the brain. In 2002, laboratories mainly used animals (primarily mice) in attempts to gain knowledge. Though helpful, mice did not have the same complexity as the human brain as demonstrated during clinical trials. Donated brains from patients helped, and eventually Brain Banks were established. These tools provided a valuable source of data, though limited.

Computer improvements allowed comparison of large amounts of data, aiding analysis, whereby particular portions of the brain could become targets (like zooming in). With continuing technology improvement, possibly other tools may become acceptable noninvasive biomarkers, which are so desperately needed.

Cerebral spinal fluid measurements of beta-amyloid and the tau protein were useful but did not seem realistic outside a clinical trial because of the invasive method.

PET scans became a valuable enhancement to the *tools* in 2004 when the FDA approval of a beta amyloid tracer (a radioactive isotope) called Pittsburg compound B (PiB) developed at the University of Pennsylvania through the leadership of geriatric psychiatrist William E. Klunk and radiochemist Chester A. Mathis.

AD blood analysis research continued without success. However, who knows what technology advancements might bring?

Genetics has benefited from technology improvements, not only in defining the first genome, but also in DNA sequencing and analysis as well as the progress made in biotechnology. (Chapter 7 will provide more information on a possible blood biomarker and genetics.)

In 2003, *vitamins* were promoted as an AD savior. Many trials were being conducted on vitamins, including vitamin C for inflammation and E for toxins, vitamins A and K for isoprenoids, fish oil and DHA as anti-inflammatory, carnitine for nerve growth factor, folate for homocysteine, and squalene for alpha-secretase. These all sounded great. After discussions with Dr. Bernick, Bruce had Ethel taking all sorts of pills, even resveratrol and a form of curcuma. Bruce stopped Ethel's pills as each trial indicated no benefits many years later. Bruce was grasping at straws and hoping for a miracle—which was not forthcoming. Bruce realized he lacked AD knowledge that contributed to pursuing these nonbeneficial promotions. However, Bruce and Ethel pursued a healthy diet. In 2002, Ethel was still doing the shopping and aware of her condition, so our diet consisted of fish, fresh vegetables (many green), and fruit with most meals, along with nuts for snacks. Blueberries and Brazil nuts had a high priority. Maintaining a healthy diet reaches a point where disease decline is weighed against enjoyment of life. Bruce's view is that this point occurs when AD decline reaches the *moderate stage.* Since damage to neurons is so significant at this stage, the patient's desires should be the priority.

Diet choices were easy as Ethel already had us eating healthy. Fruits and nuts were a norm for us as was fish ever since our days in Florida where we always had fresh fish, mainly grouper and red snapper. In California, it was fresh salmon, crab, halibut, and abalone.

During a period from 2006 through 2010, Bruce learned about clinical trials, which are covered in chapter 4. The trials emphasized the need to continue learning, both from a disease and pharmaceutical policies standpoint.

In addition to continually monitoring research on the internet, Bruce purchased *Understanding the Brain*, *Understanding Genetics*, and *Non-Fiction Writing* (DVD lessons from The Great Courses—all highly recommended.) The *Super Brain* by Dr. Tanzi and Dr. Chopra is a valuable source of information on the Brain. *Principles of Neural Science* (Fifth Edition—lead author Eric Kandel) is a valuable reference. Knowledge gained from these sources motivated Bruce to share various articles on AD and the brain with family and friends. Writing has immensely enhanced Bruce's knowledge of AD, along with improved writing skills. It is one thing to think you know something. It is another to communicate it.

Not only did these lessons provide in-depth knowledge of the brain, but they also enhanced an understanding of research abstracts, papers, and conference reports obtained through Alzforum (see Appendix B—Websites). This further stimulated Bruce to share what he learned.

Chapter 5 (The Brain), chapter 7 (The Future), and chapter 8 (Understanding AD) are results of the knowledge gained from these sources. In addition, Bruce produced a new Alzheimer's Model (Figure 2.3). A discussion of the Model follows.

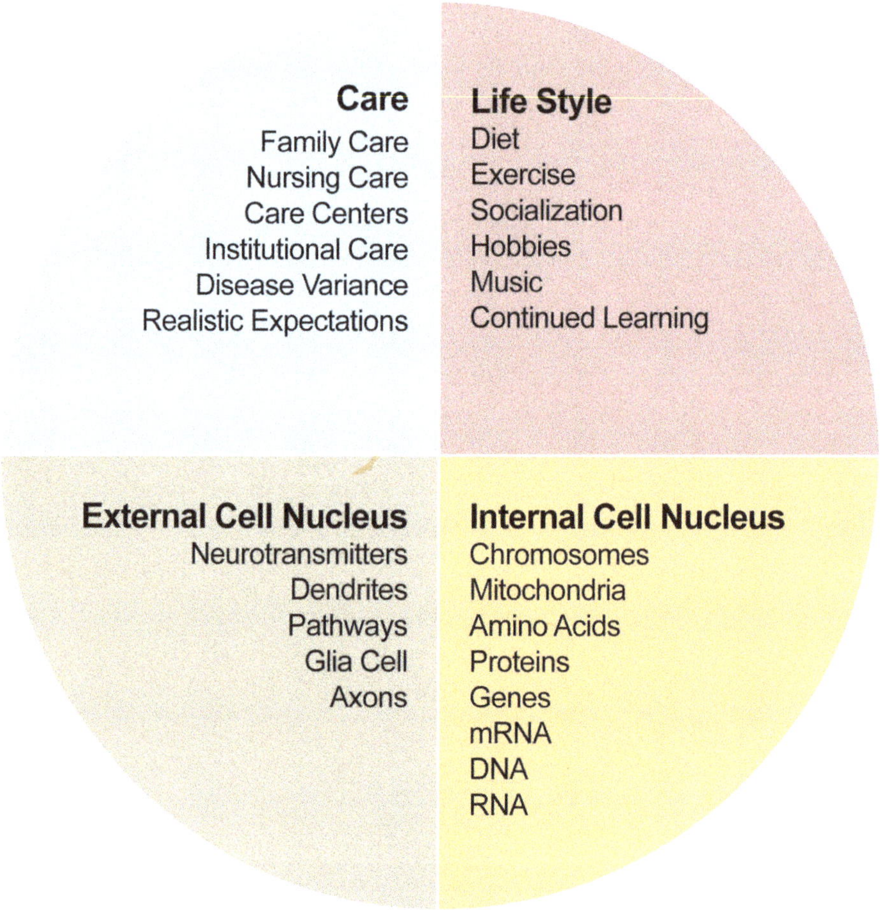

Care
Family Care
Nursing Care
Care Centers
Institutional Care
Disease Variance
Realistic Expectations

Life Style
Diet
Exercise
Socialization
Hobbies
Music
Continued Learning

External Cell Nucleus
Neurotransmitters
Dendrites
Pathways
Glia Cell
Axons

Internal Cell Nucleus
Chromosomes
Mitochondria
Amino Acids
Proteins
Genes
mRNA
DNA
RNA

Figure 2.3. Alzheimer's Model.

Since the start of the Great Society (over fifty years ago), a major attitude shift has occurred relative to medical *care*. Parents of the people who became the "greatest generation" would only consider a doctor visit as a last resort. A doctor came only if a home remedy or time could not correct the illness. Those days are gone. The "term instantaneous pill-popping society" is more likely for today's population. As with any fear or doubt, knowledge provides understanding for rational decisions. Bruce found this true for AD. At first, pill popping was our approach. With more knowledge, it became obvious that pills were not the answer. (Chapter 3—Care will discuss more caring options.)

Lifestyle is the best way to manage AD until there is approval of a delay or prevention drug, or a vaccine. Diet, as shown in Figure 2.1 (think of initial humankind's diet—fruits and nuts), regular exercise, maintaining an active social life, and continued use of your mind should become everyday routines. Ongoing education, music, reading, and hobbies should become part of a retirement plan. Use it or lose it!

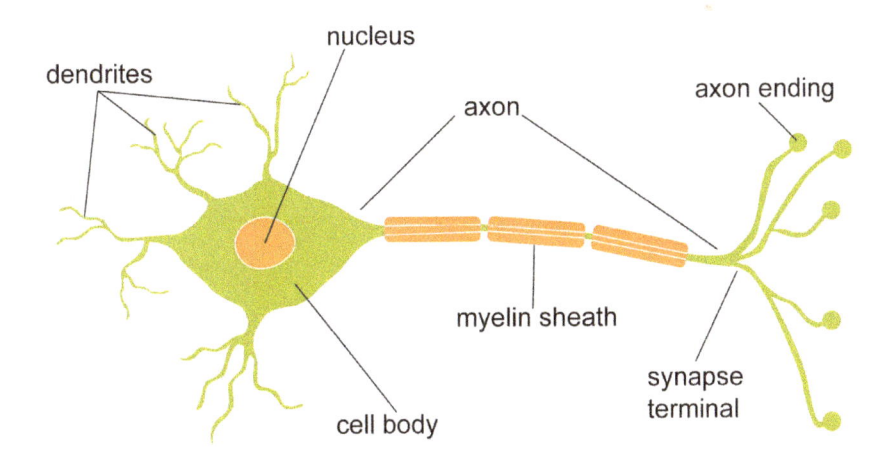

Figure 2.4. Brain Cell

The past eighteen years of research have focused on the amyloid cascade hypothesis that targets the amyloid precursor protein (APP) and the beta amyloid peptide (AB_{42}) that causes plaque. The aggregation of plaque occurs *external* to the neuron's nucleus (figure 2.4). Plaque aggregation external to the nucleus creates an assumed communication breakdown of neurotransmitters from axon or dendrites (Fig. 2.4). In addition, this breakdown becomes the predecessor to fibrils and tangles in the tau protein. A 2016 report hypothesizes that memories stored in neurons may not be lost, but only the communication links between axons and dendrites are destroyed. If proven true, a hypothesize of lost connections rather than neuron loss could open new therapeutic intervention possibilities.

With the advancements in genetics and biotechnology, research is now emphasizing the *interior* of the nucleus. Bruce views this to be the "promised land." However, as explained in more detail in chapter 7 (The Future), the challenges are tremendous. The genome's magnitude, the sequencing process, and protein creation are all complex segments by themselves. These complexities, along with the addition of understanding the brain's immune system, glial cells, and mitochondria functions, could make a realistic cure discovery more probable in decades or maybe centuries. Chapter 5 covers chromosomes, amino acids, genes, DNA, proteins, RNA, and mRNA. These are all in the *interior* of the nucleus of a neuron and form the brain's central processor.

Learn to Communicate with the Reader

The complexities of AD occur because of the magnitude of possibilities that might cause it. Scientists are dealing with a human brain that contains a hundred billion nerve cells (neurons). The complexity of these hundred billion neurons magnifies by the communication networks, where the possibilities of connections reach one hundred trillion. If this is not enough, there are five times as many glial (maintenance) cells than neurons. In addition, each neuron contains a billion subparts. Comprehending the magnitude of such numbers, combinations, and associated pathways and functions creates the difficulty researchers face.

Despite these complexities, methods of caring have advanced (both private and public). More experience has improved methods of caring. Books describing symptomatic conditions, along with dos and don'ts, have improved during the past fifty years.

Bruce's challenge to communicate with readers seem similar. Those in the medical field (primary care doctors, practitioners, nurses, hospital personnel, institutional care personnel, in-home health care personnel, politicians, lawyers, educators, and others) may find this book more relatable than the patient/caregivers who are from different countries, societies, cultures, education levels, diversities, and motivations. Photos and graphics aid through visualization. Analogy provide a relationship. Like the complexities of AD, reader communication is very difficult and there will be hits and misses. Bruce's view is that repetition is good. It is like learning anything, where practice is required.

This book does not cover the basic common-sense information contained in many current publications as well as newspapers and magazines articles. For this type of information, Bruce recommends a very easy-to-read book, *Alzheimer and Dementia, A Practical and Legal Guide for Nevada Caregivers*, by Kim Boyer, J. D. and Mary Shapiro, MSG, CMC, University of Nevada Press, updated edition, 2011.

However, attaining a comprehensive understanding of AD by medical supporters, caregivers, and family members is in its infancy at best. Can these stakeholders understand such complexity, while learning a new set of strange words and terms? This book is intended to assist these stakeholders to gain an understanding of AD, learn its medical terms, and become a reference document. Appendix A provides a list of medical words and their definitions. These words and terms become details throughout this book.

Share Benefits of Learning

When looking back to 2001 from this writing (2014–18), the learning challenge was not only for Bruce as a caregiver to increase his knowledge but also for researchers trying to understand an extremely difficult problem—AD. Just as researchers have gained a great amount of knowledge so has Bruce. The learning process motivated Bruce to share his views of Ethel's decline, along with what he learned about the disease, not only from symptoms but also from a self-educated medical study of the disease and the brain.

To appreciate and manage the disease as a caregiver, Bruce found it beneficial to gain a basic understanding of what may be occurring in the brain, how to deal with expectations, not only relative to your loved one but also relative to what your doctor is telling you, and how to understand research information that is being published. (Chapter 5 will address the brain, providing fundamentals that may help caregivers appreciate and deal with their ordeal.)

With delay and preventions, possibly decades away, and cure probably in the next century, Bruce is sharing what he has learned so others might gain knowledge, come up to speed quickly, and maintain a pragmatic outlook along with realistic expectations as research progresses.

How knowledge plays a role in fear, mistrusts, and misunderstanding, along with becoming a medical doctor, a lawyer, or a scientist illustrates its value. The doctor, lawyer, and scientist obtained knowledge and skills through education (learning) and hard work. Fear and misunderstanding can come from a lack of knowledge, or possibly the lack of effort to learn. Mistrust may be either too much or not enough knowledge. This book offers an opportunity to gain knowledge that can guide decisions, expectations, and achieve a realistic understanding of AD.

America has a reputation of being the land of opportunity. The twentieth century technological advances have changed the land of opportunity to a world of opportunity provided by the creation of the internet where learning and knowledge are attainable through a person's own effort.

Bruce found knowledge to be attainable through learning whether it is AD or any other issue. Knowledge provides the capability to discuss medical situations with doctors on their level and become part of any decision-making process. The medical profession functions on data and research that represents the overall population and tries to treat patients on how and where they might fit in that overall general data set. Bruce believes that by gaining knowledge of the medical issue you can personalize the data set to an individual's need.

Doctors who lacked specific training and knowledge of AD did not recognize that Ethel's disease started in her fifties. In hindsight, her difficulty remembering names of people at work, and forgetting conventions while playing bridge were symptoms. With continuing neuron loss, her repeating of questions became the first clue that AD could be the cause. (Chapter 3 will share Ethel's progression by stage.)

AD starts without any signs or symptoms. With one hundred billion neurons, who is going to miss a hundred thousand or so, especially since there is reserved capacity? Neurons generated at birth (a hundred billion) are what the brain has throughout life. During aging (let's use age fifty as the starting point), neurons begin dying at a rate of a hundred thousand per day. Of the hundred billion in the brain, three hundred sixty-five million neurons are lost in ten years, and almost two billion are lost in fifty years—still less than 2 percent. Bruce has not found how this rate of change varies by disease. However, less than 2 percent loss does not seem significant. It only becomes significant by considering which neurons are lost. This is evident when a stroke causes damage to a certain area of the body but not when AD starts.

The period from 2001 to 2018 has seen a tremendous promotion of Alzheimer's awareness and suggests that better lifestyle management needs to be a part of the agenda for all retired adults since the chance of AD increases with age, and cure is not a current option. Part of that lifestyle management should demand the brain to keep learning and gaining knowledge. Retirement provides time. The effective use of this time contributes to a healthy lifestyle.

Future predictions indicate that many elderly people will become Alzheimer's patients; thereby, indicating potential problems facing the United States and the need for greater funding for research. Though these predictions may truly result, Bruce offers the perspective as a caregiver that the devastating part of the disease may only last for a few years (possibly as much as three to five years). The loss of an enjoyable lifestyle does not occur until the patient's "learning and knowledge" functions are lost, and anxiety and agitation create concerns of security, fear, worry, and wandering. This probably occurs somewhere between moderately severe and severe AD and is around a MMSE score of ten or less. MMSE is a set of tests that measure the disease decline and has scores linked to stages. Normal is a score of thirty, and this score declines to zero. (Chapter 3 relates Ethel's decline by stage and MMSE score.)

Hope is eternal for all new caregivers. However, as knowledge increases through learning, realism takes over, and the caregiver recognizes that a cure is not a current option. In 2004, during a trip to St. Louis, Ethel participated in a longitudinal study at Washington University. Bruce found it hard to accept Dr. Galvin's statement that a new drug would take sixteen years from the laboratory to the market. After all, Bruce and Ethel participated in the Apollo Program where in less than ten years, a man went to the moon and returned! Dr. Galvin's comment made Bruce appreciated pharmaceuticals that receive patents for seventeen years when it possibly takes sixteen years to bring a new drug to market.

Identify "Outside the Box" Ideas

Current physical biomarkers (CSF, MRIs, PET scans) are for clinical trials but not cost effective for normal population diagnosis. An article in a 2016 *Science News for Students* presented an interesting possibility. Two sixteen-year-old (eleventh grade) students, using optical images of the eyes, measured nerve-rich fibers of the retina, the choroid artery behind the retina, and the major vein inside the retina (i.e., nerve fiber, the axon of the neuron; artery blood flow to the retina; vein blood flow from the retina). They found measurable differences in the images of Alzheimer's patients and normal volunteers. The cause of these differences is unknown. If found linked to Alzheimer's, a yearly $100 eye image could become an Alzheimer's cost-effective diagnostic biomarker. That would be great. Shall children lead us?

With technological improvements and the ever-increasing use of big data analysis, Bruce has suggested that statistical patient signature profiles be developed and used for a baseline signature if trials continue to develop criteria of mild and moderate stages for candidates. The signature profiles could utilize the past fifteen years of data collected in trials along with longitudinal data, MRIs, and compared against each number of an MMSE score. This would allow all trial volunteers to participate. With the strategic direction moving toward finding a means of prevention, the measurement criteria are even more of an issue since changes will be so small in presymptomatic candidates as well as MCI patients.

Opinions from Learning

After sixteen years of study, Bruce offers the following viewpoints:

1. Forest laboratories received FDA approval of Namenda on October 16, 2003. Its target was to excite glutamate receptors, primarily used in cognition and learning. Namenda approval stated that it includes "being a managing medication" for *moderate* and *severe* stages. Bruce found this difficult to accept after gaining knowledge of the brain and the disease. Bruce found that when Ethel reached the *moderate* and *severe* stage, cognition and learning were no longer functioning. This medication has no value to the lost neurons that caused loss of cognition and learning.

    At a cost of approximately $4,000 per year in 2015 for Namenda and $1200 per year for Galantamine (Medicare paid 70 percent), Bruce stopped the drugs for Ethel after discussion with Dr. Bernick. The expense of a nonbeneficial drug is an expense to every taxpayer when Medicare pays for the drug.
2. The 2011 paradigm shift to presymptomatic AD changed the strategy from cure to prevention. This appeared to recognize that a cure is not realistic without more data and knowledge. Therefore, finding a way to delay the disease appears to be a more realistic goal. However, the delay strategy becomes a double-edged sword. Symptomatic patients lose all hope, while presymptomatic patients who embrace risk have hope that delay could turn into prevention. The

strategy could be worthwhile if trial methods truly confirmed a delay in decline. Without improved biomarkers, will delay prove difficult to determine? When Ethel was at the *mild cognitive impairment* (MCI) stage, she went for almost seven years without significant or measurable change. Even if MRI scans indicate reduced beta-amyloid plaque, it does not mean the disease is being delayed. The AN-1792 clinical trial showed that even dissolving all plaque did not stop the disease decline. This indicated that plaque is not the direct cause of AD but has an unknown role.

3. Will clinical trials confirm a drug that can either sustain a normal balance of amyloid production with amyloid clearance or just sustain the existing out-of-balance condition? A positive answer to this question will change presymptomatic patients' hope into elation. But for symptomatic patients, without current knowledge to achieve cure, lifestyle management is the only alternative.

4. Without better biomarker accuracy, trial design and measurements become challenging and difficult to analyze due to a slow decline of the disease along with baseline differences within heterogeneous AD volunteers, and change based on each volunteer's specific parameters. Since disease decline is usually slow from MCI to *moderate* stage, presymptomatic volunteers may even be slower and drive trial lengths even longer (maybe seven to ten years) to determine efficacy versus normal disease progression. Prevention may not only delay the disease, but also delay an option for cure.

5. The need for a biomarker discovery is to find a noninvasive, incrementally determinant measurement such as blood test. Though MRIs have made tremendous analytical progress, it appears questionable as a benchmark to validate a micro change that might be occurring during the MCI or *presymptomatic* stages. Will PET scan tracer technology improvements overcome these issues?

Summary

After sixteen years of watching and evaluating Ethel's decline pattern and monitoring the clinical trial's design criteria and measuring tools used to determine efficacy, Bruce concluded that volunteer selection (from *mild* and *moderate* stages) and judgmental measuring tools used were major contributors to trial failures. Volunteers who were selected for such trials had too much neuronal loss [Ref. 16, 39] to measure change with existing tools. Even advances like MRIs, PET scans, and examining the cerebrospinal fluid (CSF) were ineffective for determining efficacy. Once the neurons are gone, there is no known recovery or replacement and decline continues. There is a hypothesis that not all neurons are used, and a reserve capacity exists.

Is it possible that in the future researchers will prove that there are reserve neurons and that technology will find methods to reconstruct pathways to restore new capabilities using these reserve neurons (like a heart bypass)? An online issue of *Nature* magazine (3/16/16) published a report by Arash Salardini of Yale School of Medicine entitled "Lost Memories Retrieved for Mice with Signs of Alzheimer's." A reprint of the article was in *Science News* (5/28/16). Dr. Salardini described how he was able to restore lost memories through a process using blue laser light. Could it be that the mice's axons (nerve fibers) were destroyed but not the neurons, and these became functional again, conducting nerve impulses as before?

Research and clinical trial tools have improved in the past sixteen years due to advances in technology. It started with the atomic force microscope, followed by magnetic resonance images (MRIs) and positron emission topography (PET) scans and improved tracers. These improved tools have benefited research, supported clinical trials, and diagnostically identified amyloid in presymptomatic candidates.

The MRI value has grown as researchers improved their ability to interpret the data these machines provided. The methodology also improved from static to dynamic or functional MRIs.

Other newly developed tracers have allowed the tau protein fibrils and tangles to be viewed in addition to identifying presymptomatic amyloid. PET scans also traced tau pathways (Ref. 47).

With the complexity facing researchers and a current delay strategy, the outlook for cure is probably decades to centuries away. So consideration should be given to provide a hospice-like environment for patients in the *moderate* and *severe* stage of the disease, minimize medications and their cost as well as allow end-of-life dignity regardless of the length of time. An alternative would be a right-to-die law for dementia patients.

Dementia

In the process of pursuing knowledge on AD, it became obvious to Bruce that other types of dementia are often confused with AD. Ethel's move to the Ronald Reagan Memory Support Suites at Las Ventanas Continuing Care Retirement Community provided a classroom experience for Bruce. Observing patients' symptoms and behavior increased his knowledge, enabling him to recognize most dementias. Symptoms observed in this small population of fourteen patients appear to indicate some to be AD patients, while others included a normal aging patient with memory impairment (a centenarian), a Lewy body dementia patient, some vascular disease dementia patients, a Parkinson's patient, a frontotemporal dementia patient (maybe with Pick disease) and other mixed dementia patients. However, this book's focus is Alzheimer's disease.

ABC'S OF ALZHEIMER'S DISEASE

The figure below illustrates the major known dementia types:

ALZHEIMER'S DISEASE AD)
Early Onset (EOAD)
Presenilin 1 & 2 Proteins

Late Onset (LOAD)
Amyloid Precursor
Protein (APP)
&
Tau
Protein

LEWY BODY (LBD)
Alpha-Synuclein
Protein

VASCULAR (VDD)
Low Blood Supply
Mini strokes
Infarcts (lesions)

FRONTOTEMPORAL (FTD)
(PICK DISEASE)
Frontal Lobe
Temporal Lobe
Tau Protein

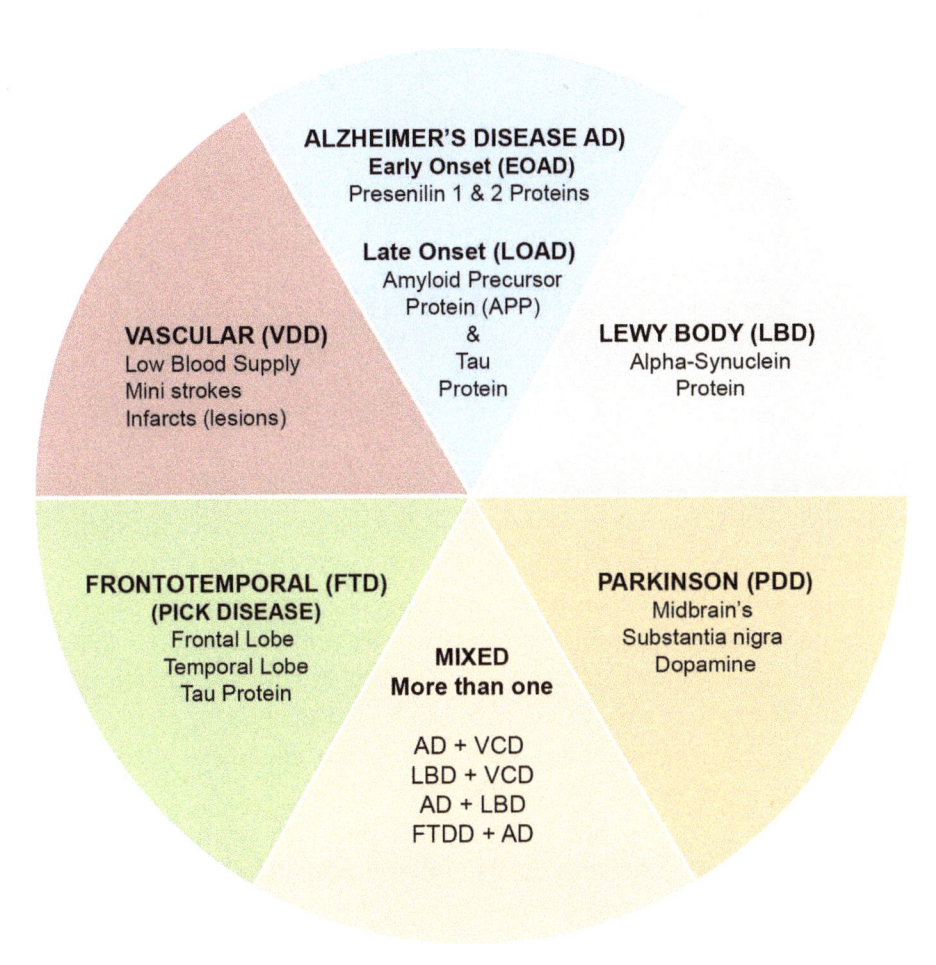

MIXED
More than one

AD + VCD
LBD + VCD
AD + LBD
FTDD + AD

PARKINSON (PDD)
Midbrain's
Substantia nigra
Dopamine

Figure 2.5. Dementia Types.

3

Caregiving

Alzheimer's disease (AD) has been historically described in three stages—mild, moderate, and severe. Caregiving varies in accordance with the progression of the disease as a patient's mental functions decline through the three stages. AD varies by individual, while caregiving varies by situation of which there are many. Caregiving issues are different for early and late AD, family situations and environment, sibling attitudes, physical conditions of the patient and/or the caregiver, financial capability, home and/or institutional care, societal diversity, government, and possibly others.

Government involvement is like a two-edge sword. Based on the complexity of AD and the demise of patients to childlike behaviors, structured protective laws for drugs, medical care, and support for those with legitimate needs are appropriate. Such care has two main options: first is a family member as caregiver; second is a home health aide or an institution as the caregiver.

The second option requires federal and state laws to assure proper care and patient protection. Health and Human Services (HHS) secretary is a responsible government department that implements federal laws. State laws vary from separate statutes for memory care or statutes under Assisted Living (AL). Nevada is under AL. Organizations that provide memory care are required to follow state and federal laws and, as such, require a doctor's order for everything they provide to a patient. State laws set requirements for the minimum ratio of caregiver staffing.

So, what is caregiving? The simple answer might be in the birth of a newborn where parents need to attend to the total needs of the baby. As the child grows, care needs are less. AD is the same, only in reverse, where care needs are less in the beginning but proceed to the stage of total care.

Therefore, caregiving skills might start by always maintaining an outward appearance that demonstrates acceptance of the disease behaviors, then always showing respect for the patients' integrity and self-ego and developing an attitude that everything is about the patient and no one else. A responsible caregiver does not focus on himself. For a husband or wife, it is the ultimate expression of love.

Caregiver's tools are sensitivity, understanding, compassion, empathy, emotional control, and whenever possible love. A caregiver's rewards are seeing patients happy, initially unconcerned about the disease and, as the disease reaches the severe stage, seeing a smile, feeling a touch, and recognition of the caregiver by the patient.

During the years of caring for Ethel (now in year seventeen), the knowledge Bruce has gained allowed him to anticipate as the disease progressed. This has been very helpful. Therefore, if caregivers could recognize cognitive and behavioral symptoms and gradual changes, they could anticipate needed care more readily. With an understanding of the brain and AD's neurodegeneration, as provided in this book, the caregiver willingly accepts the patient's condition along with discussing care with a neurologist. Since decline and symptoms vary by individual, elapsed time per stage is not predictable. Therefore, this chapter will provide Bruce's experiences and observations in caring for Ethel. The chapter will discuss *decline and symptoms* as experienced by Ethel, *home health and institutional care* experiences that will include nonverbal impacts and government influences, and, finally, *Bruce's recommendations*.

Decline and Symptoms

The disease starts without anyone knowing it. The one hundred billion neurons generated at birth are the total available in the brain throughout life. Who is going to miss a one hundred thousand or so, especially if neurons are reserved? As neuron losses accumulate, symptoms begin to appear, either during a normal aging process or as AD or dementia begins.

Originally, AD had mild, moderate, and severe stages. Mild cognitive impairment (MCI) became a recognized stage during the first decade of the twenty-first century. Presymptomatic (AD-P) was added with a paradigm shift from seeking a cure to disease delay and prevention. Others choose to define the disease in seven stages. Bruce defines Ethel's decline in six stages by having only one normal stage instead of the two normal stages.

For Ethel, the disease started unknowingly with difficulty remembering names of people at work and forgetting conventions while playing bridge during the 1990s. With continuing neuron loss, repeating questions became the first clue that AD could be the cause.

During a mild cognitive impairment (MCI) stage, pathways and nuclei damage begins to show in many ways. Repeated questions begin, and impaired multitasking begins to show, where quick decisions are not forthcoming and frustration appears.

In mild stage, damage to the entorhinal cortex has occurred (see Fig. 6.4), where pathways are lost between the hippocampus and the neocortex, which leads to difficulties such as finding a parked car (spatial episode). Eventually driving privileges are lost as agnosia (loss of knowledge) begins.

The moderate stage continues destroying long-term memory, resulting in reading and writing loss. Agitation and confusion may become more evident. The term "me and my shadow" begins because the patient lacks confidence and becomes insecure and dependent on a caregiver.

In severe stage, the inability to recall knowledge and events, along with communication, becomes impossible. Since everything is "at the moment," issues like health concerns, occupying time, diet choices, clothing selections, and feeling secure, are behaviors that are gone. During this stage, a caregiver is faced with how best to provide twenty-four-hour care for a loved one. Options include continue caregiving, hire help to assist, or transfer to a memory care facility.

Bruce is adding a post-severe stage that includes nonverbal communication. This addition shares Ethel's physical health problems and the impact of her inability to verbalize where she had pain, along with her treatment by a medical staff apparently not trained in treating patient who are nonverbal.

Aged forgetfulness refers to recall lapses such as going to find your car and having a temporary (age related) lapse of where the car is parked. Failure to focus and mentally register where you parked the car cause these lapses during normal aging. On the other hand, repetitive lapses could indicate that more serious memory issues and possibly the beginning of AD.

The slow progressive decline of the disease allows a family caregiver to become very sensitive to managing the care and lifestyle of a loved one. The first step is to accept the disease diagnosis and that AD is the cause of future behaviors and symptoms.

Alzheimer's Association Warning Signs

The Alzheimer's Association lists ten common warning signs of AD. Taken individually, these signs may mean nothing, but a person who exhibits several of them should see a physician. The tables that follow indicate which of these signs fit Ethel's decline progression.

1. Memory loss—that affects work on the job or at home.
2. Difficulty performing familiar tasks such as cooking and serving a meal.
3. Language problems, including forgetting words and garbling sentences.
4. Getting lost or forgetting what day and time it is.
5. Judgments such as dress that are noticeably wrong for the weather or the occasion.

6. Difficulty performing abstract tasks such as simple addition or subtraction.
7. Misplacing things, particularly putting objects in inappropriate places.
8. Changes and swings in mood or behavior that have no apparent cause.
9. Personality changes such as heightened anger, suspicion, fear, or withdrawal.
10. Loss of initiative, abandoning familiar interests and pursuits.

The following decline progression by stage that Ethel experienced may help as a guide for a caregiver's expectations.

Stage 1: Normal (Est. Ten Years)

Normal may sound inappropriate as a "stage," but recent research has caused this addition. A hypothesis suggests that the disease is active in a patient at least ten or twenty years before any symptoms show. This hypothesis has shifted clinical trial research focus toward delay or prevention as opposed to cure.

Ethel reflected that just prior to retiring (age fifty-five in 1993) that she had trouble at work remembering names. After retirement and moving to Sun City retirement community in Las Vegas, we played bridge. After a bridge session and unaware that Ethel had AD, Bruce would discuss conventions that Ethel missed during playing (not well accepted and, in hindsight, a bad topic by Bruce).

Stage 2: Mild Cognitive Impairment (Est. Seven Years) 2002–2008

Table 3.1. Ethel's MCI Chart

Year	2002	2003	2004	2005	2006	2007	2008
MMSE	30	30	30	29	29	28	27
Symptoms		- Memory - Spatial issues		Same as 2003 plus decline in multitasking	Same as 2005 plus noticeable stress	Same as 2006 plus language difficulties	- Same as 2007 plus misplacing things, decline in initiative
Signs		Repeat questions (locating parked car)		- Same as 2003 plus meal prep took longer, more use of recipes	- Same as 2005 plus forgot where dishes go - Guests created worry - Forgot where she put something - Wrote down for memory	Same as 2006 plus completing stories, finding words	Same as 2007 plus interest in computer games, golf, and exercise declined

Ethel displayed Alzheimer's Association warning sign numbers (1) memory loss—that affects work on the job or at home; (2) difficulty performing familiar tasks such as cooking and serving a meal; (7) misplaces things, particularly putting objects in inappropriate places; and (10) loss of initiative, abandoning familiar interests and pursuits during the MCI stage.

Though MCI can vary between individuals, it was the longest stage for Ethel. If drugs have any benefits—and it is doubtful that they do—it would be during this stage that they contributed the most toward delaying the decline process. It was 2009 before Ethel's scores fell into the mild category. Family and friends began to recognize symptoms during the MCI stage as Ethel gradually declined from 2002 through 2008. However, it did not cause any modification to our lifestyle. Most activities continued—with some degradation but not enough to prevent a still enjoyable life. We both enjoyed getting up early. During the summer, we would be at the golf shop when it opened at 6:00 a.m., where we played the back nine and then went home for breakfast, thereby beating the Las Vegas heat.

Bruce benefited and capitalized on his increased knowledge of the disease and became sensitive to most situations. Changes occurred in more ways than just the symptoms and signs. The biggest change was the recognition and acceptance of the disease. It is so common to say, "I just told you that." Bruce eliminated those words from his vocabulary. Repeating questions start out with maybe hours in between and then continue to become closer and closer to each other as memory is lost. It is vastly important for the caregiver to answer each time. *Bruce learned the importance of answering every repeated question and recognizing that each question was new to Ethel. Most difficult for Bruce was to recognize and accept behavioral changes as disease symptoms and to develop a positive reinforcing attitude.*

Symptoms and signs of decline became most noticeable in the kitchen. Since cooking and entertaining were a special part of Ethel's enjoyment, difficulties began to show in decision making of what to have for company along with meal preparation and multitasking. Planning and shopping became difficult to the point where Bruce went shopping with her. Preparing the meal became a chore as opposed to a pleasure as she worried about everything, which caused stress, frustration, and longer preparation time. One evening, veal scaloppini was the meal plan. Ethel forgot that she normally pounded the veal before cooking it, which resulted in tougher veal. Recipes and menus that she prepared from memory all her life became difficult, and referral to written aids became necessary. After working together for months (a transition period), Bruce finally took over the cooking, which eased the frustrations/agitations, and she enjoyed her new role as an adviser and helper. She always demanded that she do the dishes and clean after meals. Bruce never argued with this.

After Bruce started cooking, the change in Ethel's stress was very noticeable. She went from feeling responsible and worried to providing advice (sometimes not helpful). Ethel became more relaxed and happier during the meal. She even began eating better and more.

Once again, Ethel was very happy to entertain and have company. She would invite friends and neighbors for a Super Bowl party and have pot luck where everyone pitches in and had a great time. She would make up a Super Bowl board with one hundred squares for people to buy for twenty-five cents a square. A winner at each quarter had the score of the game at that point. At the end of the party, Ethel would say cleanup was her job, though we did it together and with the help of neighbors. During this long period of slow decline (2002–2008), it was very difficult to judge or assess decline changes as life continued normally.

Stage 3: Mild AD (Est. Three Years) 2009–2011

\multicolumn{4}{c	}{Table 3.2. Ethel's Mild AD Chart}
Year	2009	2010	2011
MMSE	21	18	16
Symptoms	Same as 2008 plus executive function knowledge loss	Same as 2009 plus executive functions, decision making	Same as 2010 plus behavior cognitive
Signs	- Stopped crossword puzzle and Sudoku - Trouble completing sentences increased	- Direction help needed - Lost interest in computer games	- *Me and My Shadow* (started) - Stopped driving

Ethel displayed Alzheimer's Association warning sign number 3) language problems, including forgetting words and garbling sentences during the mild stage.

Without an appreciation of the neuron damage when the mild stage is reached, Bruce was following Baxter's Gammagard immune globulin drug and potential trial. He liked the idea of hoping one of the drug's many unknown antibodies injected intravenously might trigger the immune system without side effect.

In September 2009, Ethel entered Baxter Pharmaceutical Gammagard Clinical Trial—*a Phase 3 Study Evaluating Safety and Effectiveness of Immune Globulin Intravenous (IGIV 10 Percent) for the Treatment of Mild to Moderate Alzheimer's.*

In September 2010, Ethel had to drop out of the trial due to an anemia problem, discovered thanks to Dr. Shin. Dr. Shin is our primary care doctor, who recognized Ethel's anemia and sent us immediately to the emergency room for a needed blood transfusion of three pints of blood with a follow-up to determine the cause—never found. Physical health became our top priority. After many months of iron tablet treatment, Ethel returned to a normal condition. A complete description of this trial is in chapter 4.

Ethel's decline pointed to a complete loss of short-term memory, indicating that the hippocampus had lost neurons and/or connecting pathways required for storing and retrieving these memory functions. A key during this phase of the disease was Ethel's ingenuity to use her work experience to help compensate for her memory problem. She would make sure she always had a pencil and paper with her. She would write herself notes as she realized that she no longer remembered things. She was using her work experience of going to meetings and taking notes. She used this technique until the disease compromised her knowledge and executive functions to where she could no longer write or even read what she wrote.

Many of Ethel's pastime enjoyments began to fade away as the disease progressed. Bruce's awareness was not keen enough at the time to discern these. Only in hindsight and reflection were these symptoms realized. Ethel would play solitaire games on the computer for hours, but that gradually faded away. She would cut crossword puzzles and sudoku from the newspaper each morning and would work them. As the disease progressed, this faded away as she became frustrated. It was so gradual that change was not obvious—especially when you are unaware that it is really a sign. Bruce continued to become more sensitive to these situations as he increased his knowledge of the disease.

Ethel's cognitive symptoms during stories of the past, along with holding a conversation, became more obvious. During these times, Ethel would have trouble grasping for the next word (aphasia) and would either look at or ask Bruce to fill in, or she would just make something up. It became obvious she had difficulty recalling past events, completing thoughts, and verbalizing sentences. However, there was no evidence of social withdrawal, moodiness, depression, or difficulty in managing money.

Ethel continued to drive during her MCI state, but during 2009 Bruce started taking charge of driving by going with Ethel to do the driving. She still drove to the hairdresser or women meetings nearby, but all trips were short and known areas. This became the forerunner to having her stop driving later. Though she was able to renew her driver's license in 2010, Ethel phased out driving in 2011. It was surprising how well she accepted it. This necessitated us to change from driving to visit the children in San Jose to flying. This created additional problems for Bruce, as he did not trust her to be alone in the airport. Bathrooms became an issue, along with security checks, personal belongings, and boarding. Each of these required special attentions. While standing in line to board a flight, Ethel set her carry-on bag down. When the line moved, she left it. Fortunately, people behind us helped. This led to Bruce using preboarding. We also learned to use family bathrooms.

Bruce's methodology of taking control of driving was to always do things together and thereby always drive. Ethel accepted this and over a period of years, it became the norm. However, it created a dependency on Bruce for everything, not just driving. This dependency evolved, and *Me and My Shadow* became included in the title of this book.

At this time, we established power of attorney for financial purposes and updated our medical power of attorney. These documents are essential, so it is best to establish them as soon as possible. Bruce recommends that these documents provide powers to more than one person.

Bruce and Ethel were now dealing with AD for ten years. Bruce gained knowledge in his role as caregiver and became more sensitive to the disease signs and symptoms, along with an awareness of future expectations. However, medical research ended the ten years with a major paradigm shift from pursuing a cure to a priority focus of delay and prevention—more in chapter 6.

Stage 4: Moderate AD (Est. Two Years) 2012–2013

	Table 3.3. Ethel's Moderate AD Chart	
Year	2012	2013
MMSE	14	13
Symptoms	Same as 2011 plus judgment, abstract thinking, behavioral (confusion, frustration)	Same as 2012 plus rational thinking loss began—long term memory loss
Signs	- Trouble using TV remote - Same clothes day after day - Bathing problems	- Family memory fading - College memory gone

Ethel displayed Alzheimer's Association warning sign numbers 5) judgments such as dress that are noticeably wrong for the weather or the occasion; 6) difficulty performing abstract thinking problems such as simple addition or subtraction during the moderate stage.

At this stage, a person is incapable of living alone. Memory is greatly reduced and knowledge loss is obvious. (Does not know day, date, time, city, state; loses ability to use the phone, TV, computer.) Aggressive and argumentative behavior may start (not seen in Ethel).

Time to Move

During our 2011 Christmas visit to San Jose, we investigated senior communities nearby the children's home as a possible relocation option. We explored a new continuing care community, under construction in Pleasanton, California. When the facility's executive director told us that Ethel would not qualify for the life-care contract, this became a trigger that it was time to make a move. In 2012, the disease was in the moderate stage and Bruce determined it was time to move to Las Ventanas, a continuing care community in Las Vegas, NV.

In April 2012, we sold our house and moved into Las Ventanas, which became our new home. The timing was right for both of us. The move eliminated dinner preparation, house maintenance, and provided structured exercise routines and social engagements, all of which made the transfer easy and acceptable.

Bruce was overwhelmed by the sensitivity of the then Las Ventanas lifestyle director (Patty Allsbrook), who immediately sensed Ethel's handicap and offered to take her to the monthly Ladies Tea. Bruce was impressed and greatly appreciated Patty's sensitivity.

After settling in our new home, exercise became a top priority as Ethel's physical capability was still very good, and she impressed everyone with athleticism. Bruce pushed a daily walk (about twenty minutes) whenever the weather was nice. Additionally, we attended one-hour strength training classes three times a week. Ethel handled these very well during this stage.

Still able to communicate and interact during meals and with a decent appetite, she was enjoying the social interaction. In the apartment, she would read the newspaper, National Geographic magazine, watch movies, and work on jigsaw puzzles.

As we met new friends, Ethel would tell them how she went to the moon—her way of telling people that she worked for NASA on the Apollo program. She would raise her hands and pull, saying she sent balloons with a camera to the moon. Each night was like meeting new people because she never remembered who we dined with previously. She walked behind me everywhere we went—*Me and My Shadow.*

Without memory, Ethel would choose the same clothes for two or three days in a row. This led Bruce to select an outfit every morning and set it where Ethel would see and use it. Bruce would leave Sunday for Ethel to select her own outfit. This worked well until decline reached the point where Sunday selections caused confusion and frustration.

Shopping for clothes became somewhat difficult as Ethel would say that she did not need any new clothes. Though she was right, Bruce talked her into some new outfits and then used the internet when needing to supplement things. Ethel's decline continued to show in activities, dining, interests, and dependence on Bruce.

Though becoming more difficult each time, we still managed to travel at Christmas to visit the families in San Jose. It became necessary to use handicap early boarding. This left the security check as the major obstacle. Bruce carried Ethel's tickets and identity material so that she would not misplace or lose them. Not all security employees were sensitive to AD.

One of the decline measures was working jigsaw puzzles. Ethel enjoyed doing five-hundred-piece jigsaw puzzles when we moved into Las Ventanas in 2012. She went to larger pieces and three hundred pieces as decline progressed. Then it was two hundred pieces, one hundred pieces, and twenty-five pieces.

Stage 5: Moderately Severe Ad (Est. 1 Year) 2014

\multicolumn{2}{c	}{Table 3.4. Ethel's Moderately Severe Chart}
Year	2014
MMSE	10
Symptoms	- Executive function (learning gone, knowledge gone) - Daytime sleeping
Signs	Ethel stopped reading newspapers and magazines, had difficulty holding a conversation, and napped during the day when not doing something.

Ethel displayed Alzheimer's Association warning sign number 4) Getting lost or forgetting what day and time it is, during the moderately severe stage.

The person that family and friends knew was now fading away. The old saying "out of sight out of mind" best describes this stage. With no memory, anyone not seen every day is soon unknown. Even though memory is gone, personality and values (good and bad) are still present. Insecurity increases (does not want to be alone). Reading becomes a problem and though Ethel tried, words failed to make sense. Sundowning (increase confusion later in the day) and wandering may start. Writing one's name becomes a problem.

In 2014 with Patty Allsbrook retired, Bruce was again impressed and fortunate to have a wonderful Las Ventanas resident, Dolores Outman, volunteered to take Ethel to the monthly Ladies Tea and include Ethel in her craft class for Assisted Living residents. This was a wonderful respite for Bruce.

Ethel's behavior became like a teenager. She no longer understood the meaning of a husband. She became very modest relative to her body. She did not want Bruce in the bathroom when she was bathing. She would lock the door. This presented the possibility of a safety issue. Bruce had all locks within the apartment removed. This incident pointed out the importance of safety concerns and aids relative to the living environment of patients with AD or any dementia. Whichever method of care, the following is suggested: (a) security code locks for external entrances; (b) contrast bright lighting; (c) clear, unobstructed pathways (avoid throw rugs); (d) locked medicine cabinets; (e) eliminate dangerous devices (knives, guns, matches, scissors, tools, etc.); (f) install grab bars; (g) use walk-in bath/showers; (h) use plastic or paper for dining.

Darcy Tumminello, RN (manager, Las Ventanas Assisted Living) was not only a venting outlet for Bruce but she also made great suggestions. She provided guidance to prepare for incontinence. Though this had not started, Bruce was trying to be ready for it. Darcy's suggestions led to protected bed covers and obtaining Depend (waterproof underpants). With Ethel not drinking enough water, Darcy suggested getting popsicles. This has worked wonderfully. She also advised that bathing could be just twice a week and that baby wipes could be used. Unfortunately, Ethel rejected using baby wipes.

As Ethel's ability to communicate declined, physical medical issues became challenging. Bruce had to be very sensitive about her discomfort and guess what might be occurring. Ethel's comment to any doctor was "I have no problems." For most issues, this was fortunately the case. At this stage, blood and urine tests become necessary as these are the best sources of information. Bruce encourages caregivers to learn to read and understand blood and urine tests.

During this period, Bruce applied the increased knowledge he acquired from The Great Courses lessons material he purchased in late 2013 and 2014. These lessons were outstanding and became a library reference source of information. He complemented these with the purchase of the fifth edition of *The Principles of Neuroscience*. These sources provided an in-depth knowledge of the brain and a valuable understanding of AD along with research abstracts, papers, and conferences obtained through Alzforum.

In May 2014, Bruce began sharing his knowledge with residents of Las Ventanas through "State of Mind" articles that were included in the community monthly newsletter. That provided the motivation to tackle this book.

Bruce's biggest disappointment as a caregiver was that previous close friends began to distance themselves from Ethel at this stage of the disease. This was an unexpected learning experience.

Stage 6: Severe AD (Est. Unknown) 2015–2017 and Beyond

Table 3.5 Ethel's Severe AD Chart			
Year	2015	2016	2017
MMSE	6	3	0
Symptoms	All prior symptoms plus behavior (changes in mood, confusion, agitation, withdrawal)	All prior symptoms plus behavior (fear, worry, wandering, depression)	- All prior symptoms plus behavior (sleep, balance, gait) - Cognitive function
Signs	- All names gone, including Bruce - Bathing became undesirable - Modesty like a teenager - Jigsaw puzzle reduced from three hundred to two hundred to one hundred	- Anger: "I want to go home." "Where do I live?" - Waking in the middle of the night, opening the door, standing in the hall	- Anxiety - Agitation - Daytime naps - Gait and balance - Meal utensil use lost

Ethel displayed Alzheimer's Association warning sign numbers 8) changes and swings in mood and behavior that have no apparent cause and 9) personality changes such as heightened anger, suspicion, fear, or withdrawal during the severe stage.

As 2015 started, Ethel reached the final stage of the disease. From here, it is variable as to how the brain and body support each other. This stage usually requires continuous care as quality of life disappears and eating, bathing, toileting, behavior control of aggression, and wandering require additional care.

With memory, knowledge, communication skills, and ability to learn all gone, Ethel's interest was only what is *"at the moment."* Therefore, as caregiver, the challenge was to figure out how to keep *"at the moment"* events and activities interesting. Without this, there was agitation, frustration, confusion, staring, and sleeping. Bruce's approach included jigsaw puzzles. However, puzzles became more difficult and frustrating as decline progressed. Bruce would then help Ethel with the jigsaw puzzle, which rekindled her interest. (Was it the puzzle or Bruce attending to her?) His approach was to help until the last few pieces, so Ethel could finish the puzzle. Ethel was very proud of completing the puzzle with no recall of any help by Bruce. Her memory was only the final few pieces, so she believed she had done the whole puzzle.

Ethel's three times a week exercise faded away as signs of potential problems with balance and interest developed. Ethel and Bruce participated in the Las Ventanas community sing-along (old songs) once a month that was very helpful. Another activity in which Ethel participated was BINGO. This was weekly, and though she did not fully understand it, she enjoyed winning.

An angel of mercy volunteered to help Ethel. Our neighbor Connie Carr took Ethel to water exercise. This happened after Bruce tried and only got her to the pool, but she would not go in the water. Connie was more successful. Connie also took Ethel once a week to play Farkle (a dice game) with a group of women.

Although "caregiving" is important for all seven stages of coping with an Alzheimer's patient, at some point in time, caregiving becomes essentially a fulltime job with associated physical and psychological challenges—not to mention the possible need for professional expertise. There is a tug-of-war between keeping a patient at home as long as possible to maintain family contact and familiar surroundings and relocating the patient to a memory care environment and letting professionals take over. This decision is monumental. Table 3.6 below provides some issues to consider.

Table 3.6. Memory Care Facility Considerations
1. Determine the level of assistance that is required, depending on the stages of the disease.
2. Address the difficulty a family has in coping with the declining capabilities of their loved one.
3. Recognize the point where it becomes apparent that an individual has problems washing, dressing, and facing the day independently.
4. Do government sponsored support group options exist and are they realistic for the situation?
5. Consider situation of spouse, siblings, sons, daughters, as caregivers—their health, availability, other family issues such as cost, living space, family/work responsibilities and relationships—and then what is best for the loved one.
6. What is the advice of the neurologist and primary care doctor?
7. Is part-time in-home care a viable option?
8. Is institutional care affordable?

Episodes

The following are some of the episodes experienced by Bruce during Ethel's severe stage before transfer to memory care.

Bras

Bruce ran into a problem of having Ethel changing her bras, so he could wash them. Ethel wanted to wear only one specific bra of the dozen she had. Therefore, we went shopping for the bra type that she likes. Women attendants at Macy's had a laugh with Bruce trying to explain what Ethel needed. Ethel became frustrated with changing bras. The attendant suggested a purchase of one bra, take it home, see if she accepts it and then buy others or return it. This worked.

Depends

In anticipation of loss of bladder control, Bruce chose to start Ethel on Depend. With help of his daughter Ann, he purchased the right size. The transfer went surprisingly well. Depend became her new daily underwear.

Bathing

Ethel's bathing was a challenge each time. Ethel desired her privacy as she no longer understood a husband, and Bruce was just a person who took care of her. On Tuesday and Friday, Ethel took a bath. Bruce started the water in the tub and placed a new Depend and bra for her to use. This worked (most times) as Ethel got into the tub, turned off the water, and closed the curtain. This allowed Bruce to enter (door locks previously dismantled) and remove the old Depend and bra. One day she was not cooperative as the Depend was not there when Bruce entered. She was standing in the bathtub still wearing her Depend. This became a difficult situation. However, after much discussion, she finally cooperated. This is the type of an episode where memory loss is an advantage. When Ethel finished her bath, she remembered nothing. However, Bruce worried about how he handled it all afternoon. As the disease progressed, bathing became more difficult. With the impact to the limbic system (memory and emotions—see figure 5.3), personality change entered the picture, and anger appeared when attempting to bathe. This required a different tactic. Bruce would first try to get her cooperation and agree to a bath. This worked sometimes, but not other times. Bruce sometimes settled for no bath and just a change of underwear. Later Bruce learned to let the patient bathe still wearing her bra and underwear.

Behaviors

As Ethel's disease declined, in addition to the above, Bruce experienced the following:

1. As the disease progresses, all reason is lost, along with the ability to communicate and express yourself. This leads to agitation and frustration along with a degree of depression.
2. Changing clothes becomes a problem. Ethel has gone to bed with her pajamas over her clothes. She sometimes says that she can go to bed as dressed and does not need to wear pajamas. Do you let her do this? How would you deal with this? Bruce used redirection. Suggest her clothes are too nice to wear to bed and she could help by wearing pajamas. Do not argue.
3. Ethel often needed specific instructions to remove her blouse or pants and put on her pajamas.
4. In the morning, the reverse occurs as she says her pajamas are OK. Still insisting on her privacy, she had worn her pants over her pajamas.
5. When not sleeping or resting, Ethel reached a point where she wanted to do something, but no longer had the capability to read, write, communicate, or maintain interest in television, jigsaw puzzles, or anything without help. This became a major increase in the caregiving time, both figuring out activities and having some personal time for myself.
6. Agitation increased as Ethel's desire to do something became unachievable. A past thought or event occurred in her brain, but the pathways to communicate or do something were lost, Ethel kept pushing for an answer. The answer did not come. Agitation leads to frustration and depression. Bruce use "hugs, hugs, and I love you" to redirect the situation. These occurrences were indicators that full-time memory care was required where trained personnel could provide activities that would keep Ethel busy all day.

7. In addition to agitation, confusion, frustration, and depression, Ethel occasionally got up during the middle of the night, got dressed, made her bed, and went out into the hall. She did not wander off, but it indicated wandering was not far off.
8. What is the impact of losing the executive function of the brain? Desire is still present, to do things and participate. Without the ability to retrieve past events, use comparisons, sentences become impossible to verbalize. Answers to "Do you like your new outfit?" could be "What new outfit?" The word *like* requires a comparison to something. Comparisons require the executive function. The result is withdrawal.
9. The disease creates the challenge for the caregiver to be sensitive and alert as well as achieving the ability to understand nonverbal communications (the sign language of AD).

So, what is it like to live with a person with no memory or knowledge of what they learned during their life? First, they are still functioning on the instinctive portion of the brain, which is in the brain stem. Though motor functions are still working, motor decline begins with balance issues along with longer time to react. Interest declines because there is no mental processing to continue progression of events as well as not being able to read. Letters of the alphabet forming words have no meaning. Names have no meaning leading to the inability to connect family members with photos.

As caregiver, it is critical to treat everything as being "at the moment" because your patient or loved one is functioning wherever his/her mind happens to be at that moment. Without memory or knowledge, there is no right or wrong. Right and wrong are learned knowledge from someone's description of a rule.

Since instinctive behavior becomes the norm, it is beneficial for a caregiver to understand the patient or loved one's value system, developed during their formative years, as these will show as decline occurs (whether good or bad). If a person was competitive, aggressive, domineering, kind, pleasing, happy, abused, dependent, leader, follower, or whatever, these valued traits will show as they are the remaining behaviors that still may be available.

At the beginning of 2016, Ethel's disease progressed to the point where she became frustrated, agitated, and anxious whenever she was not busy with something to do. Bruce judged these signs as time for either home health care services or institutional memory care.

Decision Time

The State of Nevada classifies licensed in-home care services into two categories:

- *Home Health Care Services*—Nevada's licensed home health care services provide patients with skilled nursing services, various therapeutic services, and home health Aide services *(providing the attending home health aide holds a nursing assistant certificate issued by the Nevada State Board of Nursing)*. To provide nonmedical in-home health care for clients, a home health care service must have a valid state personal care agency license.
- *Personal Care Agencies*—A Nevada personal care agency (PCA) is the equivalent to the widely used categorization: nonmedical in-home care service.

Applicants for a State of Nevada Home Health Care Services license must maintain a home office in the State of Nevada and submit proof that they carry adequate liability coverage commensurate with the range of services they plan to make available to patients.

Administrators of Nevada Home Health Care Services must meet the following requirements:

- Be a physician or registered professional nurse licensed to practice in the State of Nevada.
- Have at least one year of supervisory or administrative experience in a field related to health.

- Must appoint someone qualified and formally authorized to act in the event of their absence.
- Must attend all meetings of the home health care agency's advisory group.

Therapeutic services and required practitioner qualifications include the following:

- Professional registered nurse or practical nurse must hold a state license.
- Home health aide must hold a nursing assistant certificate issued by the Nevada State Board of Nursing.
- Physical therapist must be registered by the State of Nevada. Occupational therapist must meet the requirements of the American Occupational Therapy Association or equivalent thereof.
- Speech therapist must hold a certificate from the American Speech-Language-Hearing Association or equivalent thereof.
- Social worker must be licensed by the State of Nevada Board of Examiners for social workers in compliance with NRS 641B.
- Nutritionist must have a bachelor of science degree in either home economics or foods and nutrition or equivalent thereof.
- Inhalation therapist must be registered by the American Association of Inhalation Therapists or equivalent thereof.
- Home Health Care Agency is responsible for bonding of all staff professionals.

Personal care agencies (PCA) are different from traditional home health agencies in that they do not provide medical services or skilled services. Medicare does not pay PCAs. Many states (Nevada included) do not require personal care agencies to be licensed by the state health department. In some states a person desiring to start a business like this need only advertise, get a business license, and start hiring employees.

This is a definite "buyer beware" market. A home health care service that also provides nonmedical personal care is required to verify their personnel and accept liability for them. Personal care agencies do not have such requirements.

Home health care service is a growth industry that has developed through medical socialization introduced by President Lyndon Johnson's Great Society and implemented through a doctor's orders and Medicare or Medicaid cost reimbursements. A personal care agency is not covered by Medicare.

On January 25, 2016, Las Ventanas Continuing Care Community officially opened the Ronald Reagan Memory Support Suites (RRMSS) with sixteen independent secured units for patients. This facility was a conversion of a ground floor independent resident apartment building that contained eight apartments. The near two-million-dollar cost was resident-funded through a special project fundraiser.

With staffing in place and training completed in accordance with Best Friends' concept, the staff welcomed its first patients on February 15, 2016. The timing was perfect for Ethel's condition. After an early February physical by Dr. White (Ethel's primary care doctor) resulted in near perfect physical health, and an appointment with Dr. Bernick (Ethel's neurologist for over fifteen years) both agreed that Ethel and Bruce would both benefit from Ethel's transfer into RRMSS. Ethel's MMSE score dropped to three. On February 26, 2016, with the help of daughter Ann, Ethel moved into the RRMSS.

Memory Care Transition and Observations

The Las Ventanas RRMSS have a philosophy of having the patients out of their apartments all day as much as possible. The key then becomes to keep the patients active during the daytime and early evening. After hiring an activity director, this improved significantly.

Jigsaw puzzles are a standard. It is important to have large size pieces as well as a variety of total pieces to fit the patient's decline capability. Other activities include exercise, art, Wii, word games, bingo, music, tossing a ball, photos, along with therapy dolls and animals. Evening entertainment includes old TV programs such as *Lucy*, *Andy Griffith*, *The Golden Girls*, *Mary Tyler Moore*, movies, and others.

Ethel's major issue in transition was security. She felt very secure whenever Bruce was with her. Therefore, she had to become secure with the new people caring for her. Fortunately, the Best Friends concept does well at training personnel to create this new bond. However, it took months for Ethel to become comfortable with Bruce coming and going every day.

Diet is a difficult area for institutional care facilities, which have various constraints such as limited kitchen facilities, concerns of state inspections, and a dining manager's desire to fit everyone in the community under one daily meal plan. Meals were prepared in the main kitchen for all levels of living, including RRMSS. The RRMSS kitchen facility allowed variations to accommodate special diets or requests. Prior to Ethel's transfer, Bruce found that many small portions are more effective than one overwhelming plate. Finger foods are also more effective. Bruce convinced the cooks preparing Ethel meals to provide small separate portions. However, finger food can become toys. Dessert sweets were a big hit.

Best Friend (BF) concept and training is very effective for interpersonal daily routines. The training is evident in redirection, hugs, and conveying a loving feeling and compassion. It appeared that training in other areas could improve the BF concept. The generation gap between patient values and BF training is noticeable in areas of clothing care economies, apartment maintenance, and after-bathing maintenance.

A Mother's Day entertainment with music created a minor issue. Since music stimulates serotonin in the personality portion (amygdala) of the brain, Ethel was happy and held onto Bruce. When the music ended and it later came time for Bruce to leave, Ethel became upset. Since serotonin is associated with the amygdala, other functions were triggered including fear of Bruce leaving and the worry of who would take care of her. Redirected by a Best Friend employee, she re-established her security. Bruce's observations of other patients included a man who attempted to leave with visitors.

After reaching a MMSE score of zero in October 2016, Ethel's decline slowly continued. Dr. Bernick ordered a walker as Ethel's gait and balance became a concern. The intent was to have Ethel familiar with a walker when she needed it.

With executive function gone, the knowledge of how to use eating utensils disappeared. Ethel would stare at her food but lost the purpose of using a spoon or fork. This requires feeding her or encouraging her to use a fork or spoon. This eating issue is evident across all forms of dementia.

Ethel has now been in the RRMSS for over two years. The disease progression decline continues slowly. In hindsight, comments of worry, fear, anger, and orientation such as "I want to go home," "Will you stay with me?" "I don't have any money," and "Why are you doing that?" were transition adjustments.

During the two years in the RRMSS, music has continued to connect not only with Ethel but with most of the patients. Though a great amount of research has evaluated music effect, medical evidence is not conclusive. However, Ethel and other patients sure demonstrate a positive effect whenever they have a musical program and sing-alongs. Even as the disease progresses and decline is noticeable, music always changes the personality to a positive reaction—so much for science.

After Ethel's relocation to the RRMSS, Bruce developed his own care routine. He spent every day having lunch with Ethel. Three or four evenings a week, he took her to dinner in the main dining room, where she enjoyed the attention that she received from those who know her. She did not remember their names, but hugs and kisses were everyone's rewards. Bruce selected nights where the menu had items Ethel might eat. This stopped after a year, when the progression caused inappropriate behavioral issues. *Bruce considers the RRMSS period of their relationship comparable to their courtship period, where Bruce would pick up Ethel and they would go out for dinner or just enjoy each other's company.*

How to Explain No Memory

It is very difficult for most people to appreciate a complete loss of memory because their brains have never contemplated such. It is easy to say "Remember when" as part of a discussion without considering the answer is *no*. The following is an attempt at describing memory loss.

A simple view of a complex organ—the brain—is that it has an automatic system and an executive function system. The automatic system functions without need of the executive function such as the heart, lungs, eyes, ears, temperature control, and many others. The executive function provides all elements of learning from week twenty of gestation, through a lifetime, to a person's death. However, functions such as memory, reading, writing, perception of self, knowledge, thinking, creativity, communication, hope, desire, decision making, time, judgment, and probably others, all disappear as AD progresses.

Without storage and retrieval of events and learned knowledge, piecing together stories or relating what was learned is not possible. The written word becomes lost, as the alphabet has no meaning. The ability to sign one's name is lost. The ability to read is lost, as the letters do not register as word or names. The sensory input from the eyes and ears cannot process what they see or hear, thereby losing verbal communication. This leads to a nonverbal expression (more later).

Without past events and knowledge, the world shrinks as there are no reference points against which to gauge. The world of Alzheimer's patients becomes the environment in which they are now living, and whatever the moment is providing.

Initially, leaving Ethel to the care of the Best Friends created guilt feelings for Bruce. Guilt feelings eased with the realization that a five-second distraction eliminated me from Ethel's memory. Redirection is the key to the Best Friends care in the RRMSS.

Nonverbal Communication

Ethel's AD decline progressed to where in 2017 she could no longer verbalize her health condition or pain, except through grimaces, facial expressions, or pointing. The condition caused a very problematic and traumatic two months' experience for Ethel and Bruce.

It started on August 23, 2017, with confusion, walking, and balance problems. Suspicious of a stroke, which it was not, led to a trip to Southern Hills ER. Diagnosis was a urinary tract infection (UTI). Treatment was 500 mg of Ciprofloxacin (Cipro) and then being sent home. *This was the first impact of nonverbal communication because Ethel was unable to communicate her pain. As we learned later, the infection in the urinary tract was probably due to an abscess that was beginning on her appendix.*

A few days after starting Cipro, Ethel seem to be getting better but then declined again along with tremors in her legs and feet. *After completing the seven days of Cipro, Ethel showed no improvement.* Ethel's primary care doctor prescribed seven days on 500 mg of Ampicillin as well as a home health nurse and therapy. On September 14, 2017, three days after completing the Ampicillin and not having had a bowel movement for five days, Ethel was given MiraLAX in accordance with an "as needed" memory care order. The home health care nurse came on September 15, 2017, and recommended Ethel should go to the hospital because of an impacted colon. This time, we went to Mountain View ER where doctors determined Ethel had an *abscess on her appendix that ruptured*. A team of doctors assessed her condition and admitted her.

Dr. Nelson removed Ethel's appendix with an incision due to the abscess and cleaned the area. After surgery, Dr. Nelson confirmed that the abscess was probably the original problem and that the MiraLAX probably triggered the rupture. The Mountain View ER team ordered a CAT scan of the stomach area that determined the appendix problem. *The Southern Hills ER team assumed a UTI and looked no further. The impact of the nonverbal communication from AD and/or dementia creates uncertainty for all involved. It was obvious that many (not all) medical staff are not trained for nonverbal communication patients.*

The Mountain View Hospital attending doctor discharged Ethel on September 19, 2017. On September 22, 2017, the home health care nurse sent Ethel back to Mountain View ER with a heart rate of 149. Ethel had a blood clot in her leg that went to the lung as a pulmonary embolism. They immediately put her on heparin (blood thinner) and many other drugs as they were taking precautions. Infectious disease and hematology specialists joined the team of doctors due to concerns for a blood infection possibility. Blood culture came back negative. To prevent further clots going to the lungs and heart, Dr. Gujrathi installed a stent filter through the groin. Ethel was discharged with a prescription for Eliquis to Las Ventanas Skilled Nursing on September 28, 2017, and then back to the RRMSS on October 5, 2017.

Should the attending hospital doctor have ordered compression therapy for Ethel's legs, considering her nonverbal condition, and required skilled nursing rather than allowing her return to memory care? Was this another example of "lack of training" for demented patients?

Ethel's problems continued as her teeth were a problem as she refused dental hygiene help. So after weeks of calming down, Bruce made an appointment with an oral dental surgeon, and he removed seven of Ethel's teeth.

It is now six months later, and Ethel has made a remarkable recovery. Eliquis was stopped at the end of 2017. Though she misses her teeth, she has regained her healthy appetite. Her mood is back to her normal self. However, she has set off her bed alarm multiple times but was found unhurt on the floor.

Hospitals' Assessment

Ethel made two trips to Southern Hills emergency room (ER) and two trips to Mountain View ER, with admission to the hospital on each trip to Mountain View. The bottom line is that care depends on two issues. First is to determine the correct problem, and second is the personnel attending to the patient.

Southern Hills: The first ER trip received immediate attention. Was this due to an indication of possible stroke? Communications were very poor. The only time that a doctor appeared was at discharge. (We spent five hours in ER.) A culture of the urine was *not* ordered. Would the culture have made a difference? The doctor did not understand how to write orders required for a memory care facility and ended up doing it wrong. *Was this an example of "lack of training" for treating demented patients?*

The second trip was similar. This time the communications were with an APRN (advance practicing registered nurse) in charge of Ethel's case. Request and discussion with the ER manager was no better.

Mountain View: The first trip to the ER and admission to the hospital was very impressive. The ER doctors provided information with good explanations on each step taken in Ethel's case (especially from ER Dr. Ahmed). Explanations and offers to help came from two ER attending doctors, the head of the ER, three surgical team doctors, and the admitting doctor. The surgery team explained if and why an incision might be necessary and described the operation (this was at 11:00 p.m.). Dr. Nelson made an incision. Care after admission (on floor four) was good with continuing communication. Dr. Nelson's surgical team performance was excellent. Most nurses were good. Weaknesses were mainly in communications and roles of the attending doctor and case manager.

The second trip for the blood clot was not quite as good. Communications were not as good, both in the ER and after admission. Ethel spent over twenty-four hours in the ER halls, waiting for a room. Staffing quality was not the same on floor five as floor four. Attending doctor and case manager's experiences were not good. They were not visible unless pursued or until discharge. These were poorly appreciated roles by Bruce.

These experiences indicate that hospital personnel are aware of dementia issues but not thoroughly trained in how to treat patients who are unable to communicate. Their primary focus (probably appropriate) was on treatment orders and Ethel's surgeries. Attending doctors, nurses, CNAs, therapist, CAT scan personnel, technicians for blood, and vitals, appreciated Bruce's assistance for the nonverbal situation. How are nonverbal patients handled without such caregiver help?

Bruce found behavior of hospital personnel dependent on the individual involved, with the majority doing a very good job, but he was saddened by his observations of the RNs role. RNs seemed burdened with many administrative duties (probably connected with hospital cost recovery from Medicare) so that their expertise and time in patient care are reduced, and their trained skills are not fully used. Should hospitals have administrative personnel trained like pharmacists to manage the medical supply issues?

Therapist services appear structured to correct a body's anomalies (mainly muscle involvement) to regain normal body functions. Bruce questions whether a nonverbal patient with no memory or cognitive ability can benefit from standard therapeutic services since most therapeutic services require relearning that is no longer available to nonverbal dementia patients.

AD Concerns Facing Caregiver

- *Unawareness:* Many individuals with Alzheimer's disease are not aware they have impaired memory and thinking. Demonstrating to them that they are forgetful will not help and is likely to upset them more. In addition, partners or future caregivers may even be unaware. Awareness became a very critical issue in 2014 when a technology development (PET scan tracers) detected amyloid in the brain. Such detection, along with a hypothesis that AD begins up to twenty years before symptoms appear, could possibly provide the knowledge, whereby delay, containment, or prevention are demonstrated. This makes awareness of early amyloid detection a very intriguing and possibly difficult choice.

- *Denial:* Individuals often outwardly deny or ignore symptoms of AD but seem to be aware from their behavior that they have a problem. Research suggests that this reaction can sometimes be a self-monitoring strategy to maintain self-esteem. This becomes a very sensitive subject for a future caregiver, who recognizes the condition.
- *Secretiveness or embarrassment:* It is common for individuals to be reluctant to reveal their Alzheimer's diagnosis for fear of how others might perceive them. As a result, these individuals are often tempted to stop seeing friends or family members and become socially isolated—outcomes that are clearly undesirable since studies show that maintaining social connectedness is key to coping with the psychological impact of an AD diagnosis.
- *Relief:* Certain individuals and their loved ones report feeling relief upon hearing the diagnosis of AD. The anxiety of not knowing what is causing symptoms like forgetfulness can be a tremendous burden. A diagnosis can confirm suspicions that AD is the cause and legitimizes the need for support and therapeutic interventions.
- *A loss of self:* AD poses a threat to personality and character. Understandably, symptoms (such as forgetting faces, names, along with self-expression) can leave feelings of loss, uncertainty, and frustration.

Tips for Caregivers

- *Always answer a patient's question—each time it's asked.* It is always the first time for a person with no memory.
- *There is no right or wrong.* These are learned values that require memory and decision making, which are no longer available.
- *Normal food portions overwhelm.* Reduce food servings. Provide one item at a time with a wait between items. Do not rush. Simplify meals (use finger food).

- *Always present a positive and happy demeanor.* Remember everything is "at the moment" and nonverbal for the patient.
- *Never argue.* There is no one with whom to argue.
- *Hugs and kisses.* Positive nonverbal communication
- *Use redirection.* Manage behaviors when memory is gone.
- *Provide attention.* Just like a child, attention is a reward.
- *Use music.* Music is both soothing and can activate serotonin, which stimulates happy feelings.
- *Monitor patient's normal physical needs daily.* Appearance gives pride. Avoid uncomfortable constipation. Assure teeth and gum care. Be sensitive to mood changes as indicators of problems.
- *Always be aware of patient's Mini-Mental State Examination (MMSE) score.* Guides not only expectations but also what symptoms are occurring as the disease progresses.
- *Recognize and accept that you are dealing with the disease, not behaviors.*
- *Balance support with respect.* Consider the patient's safety, independence, and ego. This varies by stage and decline.

Table 3.7 Ethel's decline versus MMSE Scores		
Symptom/Sign	*MMSE Score*	*Stage*
Forgot person's name	30	Presymptomatic
Repeated question	30	Presymptomatic
Worked five hundred small-piece jigsaw puzzles	30	Presymptomatic
Misplaced things	30–28	MCI
Stressed by company	30–28	MCI
Speech—word finding ability (dysphasia)	30–28	MCI
Looked for car in parking lot	30–28	MCI
Performed multitasking	30–28	MCI

ABC'S OF ALZHEIMER'S DISEASE

Table 3.7 Ethel's decline versus MMSE Scores (cont.)		
Symptom/Sign	*MMSE Score*	*Stage*
Put things in the wrong place	27–25	Mild
Planned and shopped for meals	27–25	Mild
Had Slower meal preparation	27–25	Mild
Increased stress during meal preparation	26–24	Mild
Worked three hundred large-piece jigsaw puzzles	25–20	Mild
Lost interest in computer games	25–20	Mild
Stopped working crossword puzzles	25–20	Mild
Lost interest in golf and table tennis	22–18	Moderate
Stopped driving	22–18	Moderate
Short-term memory gone (Ethel would write notes)	21	Moderate
Power of attorney needed to be established	20	Moderate
Reading and writing decline was noticeable	18–16	Moderate
Insecurity—*Me and My Shadow*	16–15	Moderate
TV remote became a problem	15–14	Mod–Severe
Dressing judgment issues—help was needed	14–12	Moderate
Worked two hundred large-piece jigsaw puzzles	14–10	Moderate

Table 3.7 Ethel's decline versus MMSE Scores (cont.)		
Symptom/Sign	*MMSE Score*	*Stage*
Reproportioned meal sizes	10–6	Severe
Persuasion to bathe	10–6	Severe
Had difficulty with any puzzle	10–6	Severe
Lost interest in exercise class	10–6	Severe
Began wandering at night	10–6	Severe
Became agitated	10–6	Severe
Anxiety began	10–6	Severe
Moved Ethel to Memory Care	5 (February 2016)	Severe
Needed help bathing and dressing	5 (February 2016)	Severe
All memory completely gone	3 (April 2016)	Severe
Gait and balance declined	3 (June 2016)	Severe
Minimum assistance needed for meals	3 (August 2016)	Severe
Daytime napping	0 (October 2016)	Severe
Use of eating utensils lost	0 (November 2016)	Severe
Staring at food began	0 (December 2016)	Severe
Feeding or encouragement needed	0 (December 2016)	Severe
Fear, worry, anger	0 (February 2017)	Severe
More confusion	0 (February 2017)	Severe
Mood changes	0 (February 2017)	Severe
Balance—motor declined	0 (August 2017)	Post Severe
Help needed walking	0 (October 2017)	Post Severe
Bed alarm—found sitting on the floor	0 (February 2018)	Post Severe

SECTION 2

Alzheimer's Disease—Research

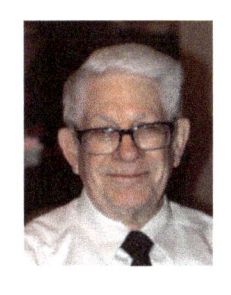

ME

MY
SHADOW

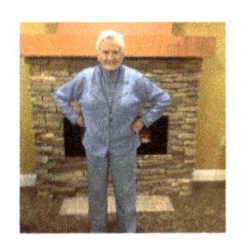

4

Clinical Trials

What is a clinical trial? Why are they needed? Why do people participate in clinical trials? Should I participate in an Alzheimer's disease (AD) clinical trial and why?

These may be some of the questions that people have facing the possibility of AD. This chapter addresses these questions and other insights to clinical trials.

A clinical trial is intended to be proof of concept for a new medical intervention (drug, vaccine, medical device, etc.) which companies (mainly pharmaceuticals) conduct based on a design protocol approved by the Federal Drug Agency (FDA). Later in this chapter, a trial protocol will be explained.

Clinical trials are normally at the expense of a pharmaceutical company that expects to recover its investment during a seventeen-year copyright protection of an FDA approved intervention. However, proof of concept requires volunteers to determine success or failure of the concept.

New interventions proceed through three separate trial phases. Phase one is to determine the safety of the intervention with a few normal volunteers. Phase two is both a safety and tolerance determination of an intervention (drug, vaccine, etc.). It often has different dose levels and monitors to determine any severe adverse event (SAE). Phase two trials have about sixty volunteers of which one-third receive a placebo. Phase three trials are large trials, some with thousands of volunteers with the disease. The trials have multiple locations and possibly multiple objectives (such as dose levels and biomarker assessment). Phase three trials usually require many years to complete (possibly five years).

Volunteers participate in clinical trials with hope and expectations that this is the intervention that will help them. Ethel volunteered for four clinical trials which Bruce explains in this chapter. Proof of concept of an intervention needs volunteers, even though the volunteer may never benefit. As Bruce explains throughout this book, the success of AD trials is limited by the complexity of the brain and the knowledge level of understanding this complexity.

Bruce's comments: *Was it possible that AD trials from 2000 did not fully assess the impact, that once a cell in the brain is lost, improvement is not realistic since neurons do not regenerate?*

Early Optimism

Optimism for a cure of Alzheimer's disease (AD) was very high in 2000, and clinical trials were accelerating as pharmaceuticals were hoping for the home run. The amyloid cascade hypothesis (chapter 6) supporters were excited by a report that Elan's AN-1792 phase one vaccine trial appeared to be very promising. In addition to the AN-1792 vaccine trial, the expectation was that by inhibiting the enzyme, gamma secretase, plaque would be prevented from aggregating and people would not get AD. Volunteers were hoping for a home run too. Caregivers and volunteers (including Bruce and Ethel) were unaware of the complexity of AD and the risks they faced.

The amyloid cascade hypothesis, proposed in the 1980s, became the guiding concept for Alzheimer's research. The hypothesis (in simple terms) is that the amyloid precursor protein (APP) produces an amyloid peptide called beta amyloid (AB_{42}). It is formed by an enzyme cutting a string of amino acids into pieces. The enzymes that are involved are beta and gamma secretase (see chapter 2, Figure

2.2). The peptide becomes toxic, aggregates into plaque, and leads to the death of neurons and, eventually, to AD. Think of the APP being a long string of beads, say five hundred beads long, and someone cuts the string at beads somewhere between number thirty-six and forty-two—creating a segment.

Bruce's hope in 2002 was for a cure. Over the next eight years, Ethel applied for four clinical trials. One was rejected because she had not declined to the mild stage. One was a longitudinal study. One was an acceptance into Eli Lilly's phase two trial of LY 430159. The last trial was Baxter's Gammagard IGIV.

During a 2002 to 2012 observation period, 413 AD trials were performed. One successful drug, Namenda, claimed delaying effects. So, why did 412 drug candidates fail? (see AD Failed Clinical Trials later in this chapter).

Bruce's Comments: The knowledge gained during 2001 to 2012 was amazing because of dedicated researchers. However, uncertainties will prevail until basic research gains the needed understanding of pathways and links between amyloid and tau as well as other areas such as mitochondria and the brain's immune system. Inhibiting gamma and beta secretase may still be a valid concept for prevention and provide hope for presymptomatic candidates.

Clinical Trial Decision

With AD having no cure and with the target now being a delay of the disease, a candidate's question is "Should I volunteer or not?" The response becomes a personal decision with no right or wrong answer. However, it is definite that for a delay or cure intervention, volunteers need to participate in clinical trials. To aid in such a decision, this chapter will (1) explain an Alzheimer's clinical trial protocol and what to expect, (2) provide research references as evidence for Bruce's views as to why so many trials failed [Ref. 27], (3) share the three trials in which Ethel participated, and (4) discuss a select group of trials.

AD Clinical Trial Overview

A clinical trial protocol defines the percentage of volunteers who participate in the drug and receive a placebo. This is a blind methodology where even the pharmaceutical investigators do not know until after the trial which volunteer received a drug or a placebo. Throughout the trial, the only indication of drug or placebo is a volunteer's own judgment or a side effect from receiving the drug. You do not want side effects. However, about a year after the trial concludes, you can make a formal request to determine what you received if you so desire. Bruce did obtain Ethel's information after Ethel's Eli Lilly trial.

At every visit, blood is tested. This is to monitor for side effects and safety. Bruce requested and received these results when Ethel participated.

Most new trials collect cerebral spinal fluid (CSF). This process is invasive and takes about twenty minutes. A large needle that draws the spinal fluid is inserted in the lower portion of the back, near the lumbar area. Ethel was kneeling over a chair-like device, where she was to "remain still." Drip, drip, drip for twenty minutes. Though invasive, it probably provides some of the best data for analyzing efficacy. CSF's AB_{42} and tau protein levels have become biomarkers for efficacy.

Also, most new trials include magnetic resonance imaging (MRI), computed tomography (CT scans), and/or positron emission tomography (PET Scans). PET scans that use radionuclide tracers—nuclear medicine.

Cognitive measurements use a variety of psychological tests, verbal response tests, and subjective caregiver tests. Most of these tests are very good for broad measurements such as changes over years. However, measurements are lacking for small, incremental changes, and these become essential for measuring presymptomatic conditions. Most of the cognitive measurements rely on subjective answers from demented volunteers or caregivers. Did inadequate cognitive measurements contribute to the 412 failed trials? Bruce believes that it had an impact.

All trials thus far used the Mini-Mental State Examination (MMSE). As indicated in chapter 3, this is a good tool for caregivers to monitor decline. MMSE scores should be requested each time a test is given, whether it be a trial or office visit.

Clinical Trials Hopes

Since there is no current cure for AD, what is there to lose? For a small group in the AN-1792 vaccine trial, the answer was their life. With Ethel, it was initially hope, but it ended up being *a significant adverse event (SAE)*.

To characterize hope, Bruce selected a current ongoing phase three trial for the drug, Crenezumab. In addition to explaining the hope, objective, and intent for Crenezumab's efficacy, a *step by step description of a protocol required for approval by the Federal Drug Agency (FDA)* follows.

Crenezumab

Accumulation of amyloid-β (Aβ) peptides and amyloid plaque deposition in the brain is postulated as a cause of Alzheimer's disease (AD). The precise pathological species of Aβ remains elusive although evidence suggests soluble oligomers may be primarily responsible for neurotoxicity. Crenezumab is a humanized anti-Aβ monoclonal IgG4 antibody that binds to multiple forms of Aβ. It has a higher affinity for aggregated forms and blocks Aβ aggregation as well as promoting disaggregation. Crenezumab unique mechanism of action, particularly regarding Aβ oligomers, provides a strong rationale for the evaluation of Crenezumab as a potential AD therapy (Ref 40).

Bruce's comments: Humanized anti-Aβ monoclonal IgG4 means the antibody is produced from human blood. Oligomer definition is in Attachment A. Disaggregation occurred in the AN-1792 vaccine trial in 2001with no beneficial effect on neurodegeneration at the mild and moderate stages. Volunteers in this trial are at earlier stages of the disease, which make this outcome of interest.

Who volunteers for a clinical trial and why? Most people (including Bruce and Ethel) *hope* the trial drug (if they get it…will they?) will delay or prevent their AD. They have no idea either during the trial or afterward whether they received the drug or a placebo. Whether they receive the drug after the trial depends on whether the pharmaceutical plans to continue tracking them in an ongoing trial. Volunteers are given a protocol of the trial. The following is an example of such protocol.

Clinical trials protocols for AD are found on the National Institute of Health (NIH) website: https://clinicaltrials.gov/search/term=alzheimer?JServSessionIdzone_ct=ktgk7i1t-b1&Term=alzheimer&submit=Search

How to use: Go to *map*, select USA, and then the state in which you live. This will display a list of trials for that state. Next, check the boxes of interest from the filters. A list of trials will appear. The following CREAD study provides a step-by-step explanation of the protocol for this trial.

Step 1: Choose the NIH trial number NCT02670083—"CREAD Study: A Study of Crenezumab Versus Placebo to Evaluate the Efficacy and Safety in Participants with Prodromal to Mild Alzheimer's Disease." (Phase three trial) (Ref. 40)

Sponsor: Hoffmann-La Roche.

Bruce's comments: The "mab" at the end of Crenezumab indicates a monoclonal antibody. Crenezumab binds multiple forms of Aβ, with higher affinity for aggregated forms, and that blocks Aβ aggregation and promotes disaggregation. (Ref. 40) *As such, it requires an intravenous injection. Sounds good—right!*

Step 2 (the Purpose): This randomized, double blind, placebo-controlled, parallel group study will evaluate the efficacy and safety of Crenezumab versus placebo in volunteers with *prodromal to mild AD.* Volunteers will be randomized 1:1 to receive either intravenous (IV) infusion of Crenezumab or placebo every 4 weeks (q4w) for 105 weeks. The final efficacy and safety assessment will be performed fifty-two weeks after the last Crenezumab dose.

Bruce's Comments: Prodromal AD means a patient is either without AD symptoms or has mild cognitive impairment. This determination is made through an amyloid PET scan or Cerebral Spinal Fluid (CSF).

Step 3: Primary outcome measures: Change from baseline to Week 105 in clinical dementia rating-sum of boxes (CDR-SB) score.

Bruce's Comments: Efficacy and safety will be determined by change over a period of just more than two years for a random group of Prodromal AD volunteers. The volunteers with MMSE scores of 30 to 22 (with symptoms) are MCI. Volunteers with MMSE score of 30 without symptoms but have amyloid are presymptomatic. CDR-SB measuring may currently be judged the best available cognitive tool available, but it is still subjective.

Step 4: Secondary outcome measures:

1. Change from baseline to week 105 in Clinical Dementia Rating-Global Score (CDR-GS) [time frame: baseline, week 105]
2. Change from baseline to week 105 in MMSE Scale Score [time frame: baseline, week 105]
3. Change from baseline to week 105 in Alzheimer's Disease Assessment Scale-Cognition 12 (ADAS-Cog-12) subscale score [time frame: baseline, week 105]
4. Time to an increase of >=4 points from baseline at any time before or on week 105 in the ADAS-Cog-13 subscale score [time frame: baseline up to week 105]
5. Change from baseline to week 105 in Alzheimer's Disease Cooperative Study–Activities of Daily Living Inventory Instrumental Subscale (ADCS-iADL) Score [time frame: baseline, week 105]
6. Change from baseline to week 105 in Alzheimer's Disease Cooperative Study–Activities of Daily Living Inventory (ADCS-ADL) total score [time frame: baseline, week 105]

7. Change from baseline to week 105 in Dependence Level Assessed from the ADCS-ADL score [time frame: baseline, week 105]
8. Change from baseline to week 105 in Functional Activities Questionnaire (FAQ) total score [time frame: baseline, week 105]
9. Change from baseline to week 105 in Neuropsychiatric Inventory Questionnaire (NPI-Q) score [time frame: baseline, week 105]
10. Change from baseline to week 105 in the Quality of Life-Alzheimer's Disease (QoL-AD) scale score [time frame: baseline, week 105]
11. Change from baseline to week 105 in the Zarit Caregiver Interview for Alzheimer's Disease (ZCI-AD) scale score [time frame: baseline, week 105]
12. Change from baseline to week 105 in European Quality of Life-5 Dimensions (EQ-5D) Questionnaire Domain scores [time frame: baseline, week 105]
13. Percentage of participants with Adverse Event (AEs) and Serious Adverse Event (SAEs) [time frame: baseline up to week 105]
14. Percentage of participants with anti-Crenezumab antibodies [time frame: baseline up to week 105]
15. Serum concentration of Crenezumab [time frame: pre-infusion (0 hour), sixty to ninety minutes post-infusion on day 1 week 1 and on week 25; weeks 5, 13, 37, 53, and 100 (infusion length = as per the Pharmacy Manual)]
16. Percentage of participants with anti-Crenezumab antibodies [time frame: baseline up to week 105]
17. Serum concentration of Crenezumab [time frame: pre-infusion (0 hour), sixty to ninety minutes post-infusion on day 1 week 1 and on week 25; weeks 5, 13, 37, 53, and 100 (infusion length = as per the Pharmacy Manual)]
18. Plasma amyloid beta (Abeta) concentrations [time frame: screening (weeks 8 to 1); day 1 week 1; weeks 5, 25, 53, and 100]

19. Change from baseline to week 105 in brain volume as determined by magnetic resonance imaging (MRI) [time frame: baseline, week 105]

Bruce's comments: Secondary outcome measures takes advantages of the trial volunteers to evaluate other cognitive tests in the biomarker tool box along with collecting plasma and MRIs to gain knowledge of Prodromal AD progression.

Step 5: Size, time, and locations

Estimated Enrollment:	750
Study Start Date:	March 2016
Estimated Study Completion Date:	July 2021
Estimated Primary Completion Date:	August 2020 (Final data collection date for primary outcome measure)
Number of Locations	284

Bruce's Comments: If successful, time to market would be mid-2022. In addition, number of locations seems high for the estimate enrollment.

Step 6: arms and interventions

ARMS	*Interventions*
Experimental: Crenezumab Participants will receive IV infusion of Crenezumab q4w for one hundred weeks.	Drug: Crenezumab Crenezumab will be administered by IV infusion q4w for one hundred weeks.

| Placebo Comparator: Placebo Participants will receive placebo q4w for one hundred weeks. | Drug: Placebo Placebo will be administered as IV infusion q4w for one hundred weeks. |

Bruce's Comments: *See Appendix A for definition of ARMS and Interventions.*

Step 7: Eligibility

Ages Eligible for Study:	Fifty years to eighty-five years (adult, senior)
Sexes Eligible for Study:	All
Accepts Healthy Volunteers:	No

Bruce's comments: Accepting volunteers at fifty years indicates pre-symptomatic condition with an identification of amyloid. Not accepting healthy volunteers indicates that healthy "at risk" candidates (those with ApoE4 gene allele and other risk genes) are excluded. Accepting healthy volunteers with at-risk conditions would provide the possibility of collecting data when amyloid first starts, along with basic normal aging data, if amyloid never starts.

Step 8: Criteria:

Inclusion Criteria:
1. Weight between 40 and 120 kilograms (Kg) inclusive
2. Availability of a person (referred to as the *caregiver*), who in the investigator's judgment has frequent and sufficient contact with the participant to be able to provide accurate information regarding the participant's cognitive and functional abilities, agrees to provide information at clinic visits (which require partner input for scale completion), signs the necessary consent form, and has sufficient cog-

nitive capacity to accurately report upon the participant's behavior and cognitive and functional abilities
3. Fluency in the language of the tests used at the study site
4. Adequate visual and auditory acuity, in the investigator's judgment, sufficient to perform the neuropsychological testing (eye glasses and hearing aids are permitted)
5. Evidence of the AD pathological process by a positive amyloid assessment either on cerebrospinal fluid (CSF) amyloid beta 1–42 levels as measured on the Elecsys beta-amyloid (1–42) test system or amyloid PET scan by qualitative read by the core/central PET laboratory
6. Demonstrated abnormal memory function at screening
7. Screening mini-mental state examination (MMSE) score of greater than or equal to twenty-two points and Clinical Dementia Rating-Global Score (CDR-GS) of 0.5 or 1.0
8. Meets National Institute on Aging/Alzheimer's Association (NIAAA) core clinical criteria for probable AD dementia or prodromal AD (consistent with the NIAAA diagnostic criteria and guidelines for mild cognitive impairment (MCI)
9. If receiving symptomatic AD medications, the dosing regimen must have been stable for three months prior to screening

Bruce's comments: Criteria determines who is accepted in a trial. MCI candidates with memory symptoms and a MMSE score of 30 may be difficult to analyze. Volunteers could remain at that level for many years. How would such stability be determined if it was normal or because of the drug? Also, what if they were placebo patients?

Step 9: Exclusion Criteria:

1. Any evidence of a condition other than AD that may affect cognition such as other dementias, stroke, brain damage, autoimmune disorders (e.g., multiple sclerosis), or infections with neurological sequelae

2. History of major psychiatric illness such as schizophrenia or major depression (if not considered in remission)
3. At risk of suicide in the opinion of the investigator
4. Presence of significant cerebral vascular pathology as assessed by MRI central reader
5. Unstable or clinically significant cardiovascular, kidney, or liver disease (e.g., myocardial infarction)
6. Uncontrolled hypertension
7. Screening hemoglobin A1c (HbA1C) >8 percent
8. Poor peripheral venous access
9. History of cancer except if considered to be cured, or if not, being actively treated with anti-cancer therapy or radiotherapy
10. Known history of severe allergic, anaphylactic, or other hypersensitivity reactions to chimeric, human, or humanized antibodies or fusion protein.

Bruce's summary comments for the Crenezumab trial:

1. *Volunteers should request assurance of participating in an open label trial upon completion of their participation. This provides a bridge from a successful trial until the market is available.*
2. *Volunteers should understand what is involved with an amyloid PET scan, cerebral spinal fluid collection, and data they can receive and data they cannot receive and why.*
3. *Volunteers should request the protocol to identify specific action that the trial sponsors take, if a Severe Adverse Event (SAE) occurs and how they determine such an event.*
4. *Potential questionable issues:*
    (a) *CDR-SB validation was based on mostly demented subjective data. How will CDR-SB measure very small changes in presymptomatic volunteers?*
    (b) *Is two years enough time for volunteers with MMSE score of 30 (either with or without symptoms) to have*

measurable changes? (see Table 3.1 for Ethel MMSE score between 2002 and 2005)

(c) *Why weren't amyloid PET scans used to measure changes in amyloid along with tau PET scan to detect entorhinal cortex (EC) impact? (Discussed in chapter 6.)*

5. Secondary trial measure should provide valuable data on pre-symptomatic progression.

AD Failed Clinical Trials

"Alzheimer's disease drug-development pipeline: few candidates, frequent failures," Jeffrey L Cummings et al. [Ref 27] indicated one successful trial and 412 failed unique compounds, for which only eighty-three phase three trials were conducted. A simple answer for failed trials could be the complexity of the disease and brain. However, further assessments suggest alternative views. Pharmaceutical companies continue to hope the next drug will be the home run. The depth of knowledge of the brain's functions, processes, and sophistications is only in its infancy. What is not known appears to be far greater than what is known.

Most AD knowledge has come from autopsies up to the start of the twenty-first century. Late twentieth century technology has provided tools to advance the knowledge base and support clinical trial investigations. A question for trial sponsors is "How was/is past research evidence weighed in formulating clinical design criteria?"

Was there a flaw in failed trials, the acceptance of volunteers with mild and moderate AD? Have volunteers in the mild and moderate stages of AD already lost too many irreplaceable neurons to show any improvement? Mild and moderate stage patients' symptoms include loss of short-term memory (hippocampus) and executive functions (neocortex). The entorhinal cortex (EC) plays a crucial role as a gateway connecting the neocortex and the hippocampal formation. [Refs. 16] Late twentieth century evidence [Refs. 16 & 39] indicated the EC had significant damage in the very early mild stage of AD. Chapter 6 will describe this evidence.

Was another trial flaw in the measuring tools used to determine change? Though the tests were the best available, they were and still are subjective assessments. Such assessments include uncertainties. Mathematics and statistics may apply justifications to minimize these uncertainties. However, if this is acceptable reasoning, then the same rational justification should apply to the creation of a signature profile to be used as a placebo signature, thereby having all patients receiving the drug.

After sixteen years of study, Bruce offers his views for failed trials: (a) depth of research knowledge was either insufficient or not totally accepted, (b) cognitive measuring tools were the best available but questionable and debatably inadequate, (c) design criteria specified only mild and moderate stage candidates; unknowingly these volunteers were too far demented to demonstrate efficacy, (d) a requirement demonstrating disease improvement was not attainable based on the volunteers' decline status, (e) leadership was lacking to provide organization and a systematic AD approach. However, knowledge increased, and recognition of the deficiencies influenced a strategic change from targeting cure to pursuing interventions for prevention, effective treatment, and delay of the AD and related dementia (ADRD).

Ethel's Four Clinical Trials

In 2002, we applied for a gamma secretase trial being conducted in San Diego, but Ethel was rejected because she scored too high for the trial design criteria which was for mild and moderate patients. The gamma secretase trial itself failed. As indicated above, perhaps this trial failure was due to the wrong criteria for accepting volunteers. Possibly, Ethel was the right candidate.

It was during a 2004 visit to St. Louis that Ethel entered a longitudinal study at Washington University. In addition to MMSE and physiological testing, Dr. Bateman did an MRI scan (this was the infancy of MRI analysis). Dr. Allison Goethe conducted a spinal tap to collect spinal fluid. After all the tests were completed, we met with Dr. Galvin who stated Ethel had mild cognitive impairment (MCI), which we already knew. However, in discussion with him about research, he said, "From the time a pharmaceutical company starts a new drug development, and if successful, it would take sixteen years to reach the market." This was astonishing information and hard to believe. We soon learned the value of the information provided by Dr. Galvin.

It was 2006, and Ethel was at a borderline between MCI and mild Alzheimer's disease. Somehow, she was accepted to participate in Eli Lilly's LY450139 phase two trial described as follows:

ClinicalTrials.gov Identifier: NCT00244322: Effects of LY450139 Dihydrate on Subjects with Mild to Moderate Alzheimer's Disease.

Sponsor: Eli Lilly. First received: October 24, 2005.

Purposes: Determine the safety of LY450139 dihydrate and any side effects that might be associated with it. How much LY450139 dihydrate should be given, and how long it may be detected in blood. Determine if LY450139 dihydrate may affect a peptide found in blood, called abeta. This peptide is studied in subjects with AD. Collect and store samples from blood and spinal fluid for research related to AD and similar (neurodegenerative) diseases or inflammation (irritation) that may provide information on how subjects respond to LY450139 or other medications.

Primary Outcome Measures: Safety and tolerability.

Secondary Outcome Measures: Determine levels of peptides in blood and spinal fluid that might relate to AD. Evaluate changes in thinking and memory. Evaluate changes in daily living activities. Determine levels of study drug in blood and spinal fluid.

Results: Group differences were seen in skin and subcutaneous tissue complaints (P = 0.052). These included three possible drug rashes and three reports of hair color change in the treatment groups. There were three adverse-event-related discontinuations, including one report of transient bowel obstruction.

Plasma *Aβ40* was reduced by 58.2 percent for the 100 mg group and 64.6 percent for the 140 mg group (P<0.001). No significant reduction was seen in CSF *Aβ*. No group differences were seen in cognitive or functional measures.

Conclusions: LY450139 was generally well tolerated at doses of up to 140 mg taken daily for fourteen weeks, with several findings indicating the need for close clinical monitoring in future studies. Decreases in plasma Aβ concentrations were consistent with inhibition of γ-secretase.

This six-month trial was being conducted at the University of California, San Diego (UCSD) in La Jolla, California, which was three hundred miles from our home in Las Vegas, Nevada. The trial required a trip every other week. We would leave Las Vegas at 5:30 a.m. every other Wednesday and return home about 6:30 p.m. We stayed overnight the first and last trips plus two other trips as they collected spinal fluid on those trips. Ethel thought whatever she was taking was doing some good.

Years later, Bruce received confirmation from Dr. Siemers (Eli Lilly's principal investigator—PI) that Ethel received the high drug dose. However, Dr. Siemers *rejected Bruce's inquiry for an open label participation in the following phase three trial.* When Eli Lilly started the phase three trial, they retitled LY-450139 to semagacestat. Eli Lilly's phase three semagacestat data indicated some delay progress on volunteers with high mild scores (MMSE 26*)*. Volunteers who completed the phase three trial continued participation in an open-label trial segment that assured receiving the drug. *It was unfortunate for Ethel as well as Dr. Siemers, that he did not have the foresight to follow the phase two patients in an open label segment of the phase three.* There were indications (2015) that Eli Lilly might pursue semagacestat for MCI and presymptomatic patients.

Semagacestat (LY450139) is a gamma-secretase inhibitor which lowers β-amyloid in blood and spinal fluid in humans tested thus far and in blood, spinal fluid, and brain in animals tested thus far. The phase three trial used several different tests to measure the effect of semagacestat on both β-amyloid and amyloid plaques for some volunteers. The build-up of amyloid plaques was measured by a brain scan that takes a picture of amyloid plaques in the brain. Other tests measured the overall function of the brain and brain size in some participants.

Bruce's Comments: Results: Plasma Aβ40 was reduced by 64.6 percent for the 140 mg group. Ethel received the 140 mg, and said she thought it helped. Ethel was marginable for acceptance with MMSE 27. She probably benefited from this drug. However, trial measurements did not indicate any benefits. (No group differences were seen in cognitive or functional measures.) Could it have been that the drug was effective for Ethel at her early stage, but due to the mild and moderate selection criteria and test measuring tools, the overall population results hide any benefits for early stage volunteers?

As Bruce gained knowledge, he developed the opinion that failed clinical trials did not necessarily show that drugs were not beneficial, but that the tools to measure the degree of change in trial volunteers were inadequate. The possible small benefits experienced by early stage patients were never isolated but were included in the overall trial population where such grouping could not meet trial design criteria.

Without the appreciation of neuron damage when the mild stage is reached, Bruce was following Baxter's Gamma Gard immune globulin drug and potential trial. He liked the idea of hoping one of the drug's many unknown antibodies injected intravenously might trigger the immune system without side effect. In late September 2009, Ethel enrolled in Baxter Pharmaceutical Gammagard Clinical Trial—*A Phase Three Study Evaluating Safety and Effectiveness of Immune Globulin Intravenous (IGIV 10 Percent) for the Treatment of Mild-to-Moderate Alzheimer's. (ClinicalTrials.gov—Identifier: NCT00818662).* Ethel received MRIs in October 2009 and other tests at the start of the trial. Then every two weeks a nurse would come to the house and start an intravenous injection. This would drip into Ethel's system and usually take about an hour. Every three months, she had a checkup that included blood work, tests, and an MRI.

Ethel's Anemia Issues

Sometime during July, August and September of 2010, Ethel apparently developed either one or multiple ulcers in her colon. The ulcers appear to have led to a slow blood loss over an unknown period. Ethel's AD masked her awareness of this condition. Ethel was unable to recognize or explain any problem. External symptoms might have been evident to a professional, if Ethel or Bruce could have communicated effectively. However, the professional nurses performing the bi-weekly infusions failed to detect any obvious signs.

Signs that might have been evident in hindsight (Monday morning quarterbacking) were Ethel said she was cold very often. Ethel slept a lot during the day. Ethel had bowel issues for which she used pads to absorb what she called squirting (may have been liquid caused from the bleeding). Ethel became unsteady during the period (probably light headed from blood loss). Ethel's skin was pale.

A September 22, 2010, blood test indicated an alarming hemoglobin count of 7.7 g/dl initiating a concern of anemia. Ethel and Bruce were unfortunately traveling. They did not find out about the problem until September 27, 2010. They returned immediately on September 28, 2010, and saw Dr. Shin, who directed Ethel to the hospital ER on September 29 after an exam indicated blood in the stool. Ethel's hemoglobin count was 6.8 g/dl in the ER. A transfusion of three units of blood was started and Ethel was admitted to the hospital. Ethel's hemoglobin count increased to a normal 11.8 g/dl after completing the blood transfusion on September 30, 2010. After an exam indicated blood in the stool, the hospital wanted to do an immediate colonoscopy. Bruce said no to this and arranged for her gastrologist to do this. She was released from the hospital after a colonoscopy, and upper GI tests were scheduled with Dr. Gitlin for October 6, 2010.

Dr. Gitlin found healing ulcers in the beginning of the colon. An upper GI test result was normal. Dr. Gitlin's findings indicated ischemic colitis and collagenous colitis (inflammatory colon disease—watery diarrhea).

On October 12, 2010, Charina Toste, APN ordered blood work. On October 27, 2010, Charina Toste determined that Ethel's anemia was resolved but she had an iron deficiency from the blood loss. She hypothesized that the cause of the iron deficiency anemia was the ulcers that were healing in the colon. She prescribed ferrous sulfate 325 mg capsules to be taken on Saturday and Sunday. She indicated that Ethel's iron should be normal in a couple of months. Ethel's clinical trial infusions had been put on hold because of this event. All drugs except Lexapro and Alendronate were stopped. Neither the hematologist nor the doctors expressed any concern for the change in lymphocytes after the blood transfusion. Blood results were acceptable on January 17, 2011, but lower than when the trial started. An iron deficiency was still present. Ethel was back to normal by April 2011. This was our last clinical trial.

The doctors could only assume that the healing ulcers were the cause of an iron deficiency anemia. The cause for the ulcers is unknown. Infection, inflammation, drug interaction, and trial infusions were all possibilities. It appears that the body immune system resolved the problem with help from the blood transfusion. Ethel's elimination system has been problematic for a long time. She has had constipation and/or diarrhea problems for years. This condition, along with drug side effects, might have produced inflammation that caused colon ulcers. Collagenous colitis identified above probably played a role.

A request was made to stop Ethel's trial participation and unblind her data to confirm whether she was getting the drug or a placebo (data suggest drug). Principal investigator (Dr. Relkin) suggested a trial hold for Ethel until cause was determined. (*Infusions were stopped*, and Ethel withdrew from the trial.)

Though reported to Baxter, it is not known whether this was described as a significant adverse event (SAE) because feedback was never received. Bruce believes it certainly should have been documented as such.

This trial completed in 2012. Baxter initiated a follow-up larger trial (ClinicalTrials.gov Identifier: NCT01736579) in 2012, which was terminated in 2015 as not achieving the trial's end-point criteria.

AD Clinical Trials of Interest

The first transgenic mouse model in 1995 provided research laboratories a tool to conceive, design, and test clinical trials concepts. The initial approach was for a beta amyloid peptide vaccine. Next was for monoclonal antibodies targeting gamma secretase, and finally a trial concept for Prodromal AD (presymptomatic volunteers with confirmed amyloid). Discussion of these three approaches follow relative to their clinical trials.

AD Vaccine Trial (AN-1792)

It was 2001, and Bruce's school of the future began like a roller coaster, with ups and downs as well as twists and turns. After successful laboratory transgenic mouse trials, ELAN Pharmaceutical phase one study brought excitement when it showed positive results for the Vaccine AN-1792. However, the elation at the top of the roller coaster came crashing down with a sinking feeling in the stomach as the phase two-a trial terminated in February 2002.

Vaccines were successful with such diseases as polio, tuberculosis, scarlet fever, and others. However, AN-1792 vaccine was too early for AD because of the need for more knowledge about the mechanisms of the brain's immune system.

AN-1792 was the first active immunotherapy strategy for Alzheimer's disease. *The rationale was that AN-1792 would induce an immune response that would remove brain amyloid deposition.* Extensive preclinical animal evidence showed that immunization with $A\beta 1\text{-}42$ peptide could prevent or reverse the development of the neuropathological hallmarks of AD, including amyloid plaque formation, neurotic dystrophy, synaptic loss, gliosis, and impaired performance in behavioral assays. (Ref. 1)

AN-1792 was the name for a vaccine that was under investigation for its potential to stimulate the immune system to *recognize* and attack the amyloid plaque that was hypothesized as a hallmark of AD. The drug, commonly known as the *Alzheimer's vaccine*, was a synthetic beta-amyloid peptide (AB42). A peptide is a small segment of less than fifty amino acids. Scientists at Elan Corporation developed the treatment based on the theory that administration of beta-amyloid peptide would activate the brain's immune system to produce its own anti-amyloid antibodies, thereby clearing the beta-amyloid plaque. Research and development of AN-1792 was conducted as a collaborative effort by Elan and Wyeth-Ayerst Laboratories, the pharmaceutical division of American Home Products.

Findings reported in the July 1999 issue of *Nature* [Ref. 1] raised tantalizing possibilities of using vaccinations to prevent or ameliorate AD. A study by Dale Schenk and colleagues at Elan Pharmaceuticals reported that PDAPP transgenic mice (their genes modified by biotechnology) were immunized with synthetic $A\beta_{42}$. The findings, while intriguing, were just a first step. Many questions and problems had to be addressed before an Alzheimer's vaccine could be considered. The transgenic mouse models were an incomplete model of the human disease. While the mice accumulated amyloid in their brains, they did not display the behavioral, histological, or physiological defects seen in human AD. Moreover, as Peter St George-Hyslop and David Westaway pointed out, it was not yet (1999) known whether *extracellular Aβ deposits* were causing neuronal dysfunction and death or were merely a consequence of the disease. What the study offered was another method by which to test the critical beta-amyloid hypothesis.

Based on these preclinical results, both the U.S. Food and Drug Administration (FDA) and the U.K. Medicines Control Agency permitted phase one human trials of AN-1792 to assess its safety and tolerability in people with mild to moderate Alzheimer's disease. The trial enrolled eighty volunteers.

Results from the phase one trial were announced in 2000 and suggested the vaccine was well tolerated in human recipients. Tests also showed that some volunteers developed anti-amyloid antibodies. Based on these outcomes, Elan began planning a phase two-a trial in the United States and Europe for late 2001.

A follow-up of the September 2000 AN-1792 phase one trial was conducted from June of 2003 to September 2006. [Ref. 18] During the six years from the start of AN-1792 phase one, forty-two of the eighty volunteers died—twenty of them before the start of the June 2003 follow-up trial. Eight of the twenty volunteers who died had received the drug and committed their brains to postmortem examination.

Reported significant findings were: AN-1792 AB vaccine triggered the immune system that cleared beta amyloid plaque from the neocortex. Seven of eight immunized volunteers who underwent postmortem assessments, including those with virtually complete plaque removal, had severe end-stage dementia before death. (Ref. 18)

For the group receiving the AN-1792 vaccine versus the placebo group, no evidence was found to indicate end-of-life survival improvement or of an improvement in the time span leading to severe dementia.

Bruce's phase one comments: *Although immunization with amyloid beta resulted in reported clearance of amyloid plaques in volunteers with AD, plaque removal did not prevent progressive neurodegeneration. If clearing plaque was successful but the disease continues with no difference to the end of survival, this seems to indicate that plaque may not be a cause of the disease but may be just a contributor of some sort*

In August 2001, AN-1792 the phase two–a clinical trial named Randomized Safety, Tolerability, and Pilot Efficacy of AN-1792 in Alzheimer's Disease—was initiated with an enrollment of 370 volunteers with mild to moderate AD at investigational sites in the United States and Europe. Approximately three hundred volunteers were randomly selected to receive AN-1792 vaccine, and the rest received a placebo (inactive treatment). Patients were evaluated using standard current clinical assessments of cognition and memory. A goal of the study was to evaluate the clinical impact of eliciting an immune response (formation of antibodies) to the A-beta peptide in patients with AD.

Elan Corporation announced January 17, 2002, that it would suspend further drug administration in the phase two-a clinical trial of its therapeutic vaccine AN-1792, made of synthetic $A\beta 1$-42 peptide. (Ref. 3) Four volunteers had fallen ill with what appeared to be central nervous system inflammation. On February 22, 2002, an additional twelve volunteers were added to the previous four. (Ref. 4) A safety committee terminated the AN-1792 phase two-a trial at the end of February 2002.

Eighteen of three hundred (or 6 percent) of the volunteers who had received the vaccine were reported to have meningoencephalitis at the time the trial was terminated. Most volunteers, but not all, were successfully treated. (See Appendix D for a case study and explanation.)

At the time the trial terminated, two volunteers had received one injection, 274 volunteers had received two injections, and twenty-four volunteers had received three injections. Of the three hundred AN1792 treated volunteers, fifty-nine (19.7 percent) developed the anticipated immune system antibody response.

After the trial termination, there were varied reports on cognitive improvement for those who generated an antibody response to the vaccine (responders). There were claims of improvement based on trial tests and measurements of antibody responder's ability to maintain a functional home, lifestyle, and environment, along with caregiver observations. (Ref. 8) Other reports indicated the contrary. Significant differences were not found between antibody responders and the placebo group for ADAS-Cog, Disability Assessment for Dementia, Clinical Dementia Rating, MMSE, or Clinical Global Impression of Change. (Ref. 11) A small subset of volunteers had cerebral spinal fluid (CSF) examinations. Reports indicated that tau in the CSF decreased in antibody responders. (Ref. 11)

Cognitive test methods and tools are called into question, with some reports citing cognitive improvements and other reports stating that no cognitive differences were found. (Ref. 11) *The need for nonjudgmental biomarkers is critical.*

One hundred and fifty-nine volunteers/caregivers (thirty placebo and 129 AN-1792) participated in this AN-1792 follow-up study (Ref. 15) from January to October 2006. Of the one hundred twenty-nine treated volunteers, twenty-five were antibody responders. Of these twenty-five, nineteen were able to provide test samples. Seventeen of the nineteen showed low but detectable anti-AN-1792 titers—lab tests that measure antibodies. (This was nearly five years later.) The 104 volunteers, who received the AN-1792 vaccine but did not develop immune system response from the vaccine, remained without detectable antibodies.

The Disability Assessment for Dementia (DAD) scale tests indicated less decline among antibody responders compared to placebo-treated volunteers after 4.6 years (See Appendix B, Websites for DAD description). The Dependence Scale (See Appendix B, Websites for description) also indicated that antibody responders showed significantly favorable differences. Of a small number of volunteers who underwent a follow-up MRI, antibody responders showed similar brain volume loss during the follow-up period compared with placebo-treated volunteers. (Ref. 15, Ref. 17)

Greenberg and colleagues suggested that the vaccination may have triggered an inflammatory response against amyloid in the blood vessels, resulting in abnormal cerebral blood flow that was responsible for clinical decline. (Ref. 6)

Bruce's Comments: A hindsight question is, "Would this trial have been started if the knowledge from the AN-1792 phase one follow-up trial ending in 2006 had been available?" Unanswered questions include (1) Antibody responders' autopsied brains showed all plaque removed—so what caused continuation of the disease? (2) Why did the disease continue at the same rate for both antibody responders and placebo volunteers if plaque caused AD? (3) What caused some volunteers to be responders and others who received the vaccine to not respond?

Based on the impact from the failed vaccine trial, a switch was made to monoclonal antibodies which are recognize by a drug name ending in "mab."

A monoclonal antibody is designed to bind to a specific target such as plaque (AB_{42}) or soluble amyloid peptide (AB_{40}) or a subelement of a peptide (oligomers).

The antibody design may be for removal of excess quantities of the beta amyloid or inhibit overproduction. Though conceptually logical, trials with mild and moderate AD volunteers proved unwise as their disease progressed too far. These trials included bapineuzumab, gantenerumab, crenezumab, aducanumab, and solanezumab. Some antibody drugs are testing pre-symptomatic and MCI volunteers.

Bruce's Comments: These drugs may prove useful for pre-symptomatic volunteers by delaying the disease progress if provided at the right stage of the disease. The A4 trial's following discussion is currently testing Solanezumab.

A4 Trial—Solanezumab

The Clinical Trial of Solanezumab for Older Individuals Who May be at Risk for Memory Loss (A4) (NCT02008357) started in 2014 and involves 1,150 volunteers at sixty locations in Australia, Canada, Japan, and the United States, including the Cleveland Clinic in Las Vegas. It is a collaborative sponsorship by Eli Lilly and Alzheimer's Therapeutic Research Institute (with significant private and public funding). A target completion is July 2022.

A strategy redirection toward prevention/delay occurred in 2011 based on the acceptance that volunteers in the Mild and Moderate stages have lost too many neurons. Using PET scans with tracers that identified amyloid, scientists confirmed during 2012 and 2013 that amyloid appears in people in their late forties and early fifties. These findings, along with analysis of data from ADNI and AIBL, guided the selection criteria used in the A4 trial design. ADNI and AIBL are discussed below.

TheA4 trial is significant because its design was predicated on lessons learned from failed trials as well as from research efforts during 2012 and 2013 to upgrade cognitive biomarkers to be used and to establish baseline criteria for selecting candidates without symptoms.

The A4 clinical trial increased the initial design from 168 to 240 weeks along with a Solanezumab dose increase from 400 mg to 1600 mg [Ref. 48]. A new end date of July 2022 was established for this placebo-controlled secondary prevention trial of an anti-Aβ treatment, aimed at slowing cognitive decline in cognitively normal older individuals who have elevated brain amyloid levels (i.e., Aβ-positive individuals) based on the tracer, Florbetapir and PET amyloid imaging. Evidence has shown elevated amyloid levels to be precursors of AD and other cognitive diseases.

Two desirable capabilities lacking during the decade of failed trials were linking cognitive markers to clinical markers (i.e., verbal subjective tests vs. imaging/CSF tests) and lacking sensitivity measurements for small incremental changes. A research report, The Preclinical Alzheimer Cognitive Composite: Measuring Amyloid-Related Decline by Michael C. Donohue et al, August 3, 2014, states, "We must develop outcome measures sensitive to the earliest disease-related changes" and then describes the methods for intervention in the presymptomatic phases of the disease.

The Alzheimer Disease Cooperative Study Preclinical Alzheimer Cognitive Composite (ADCS-PACC) is the result of 2012/2013 research to upgrade cognitive measurements and prove biomarker efficacy during the A4 clinical trial.

ADCS-PACC includes a composite of four measures: (1) The total recall score from the Free and Cued Selective Reminding Test (FCSRT) (zero to forty-eight words), (2) the delayed recall score on the Logical Memory II-a subtest from the Wechsler Memory Scale (zero to twenty-five story units), (3) The Digit Symbol Substitution Test score from the Wechsler Adult Intelligence Scale—Revised (zero to ninety-three symbols), and (4) The MMSE total score (0–30 points).

The A4 trial is the most promising AD study in the past twenty years. Could Solanezumab be the AD equivalent to cardiac disease statins? The trial is not without issues—disclosure of the disease to volunteers being one, along with public/private joint funding. Though it does not benefit symptomatic patients, it may benefit future generations. In addition, knowledge gained from the asymptomatic (AB negative—noncarriers) volunteers could be huge in comparative analysis. Finally, perhaps the small incremental progression change would provide data for a future "signature profile" that could eliminate placebo needs.

Bruce has been following this monoclonal antibody (MAB) since its basic laboratory beginning at Washington University (St. Louis) in March 2001 and its phase three efficacy failure in 2009.

After a failure, why start a new A4 trial? Mild and moderate stage volunteers of the failed trials were at the wrong stages and having too many neurons already lost. The A4 trial's hope is to show efficacy by slowing the disease that has not reached the stage of symptomatic damage—thereby, clearing soluble amyloid and preventing plaque formation and the initiation of the hypothesized cascade to a loss of neurons. Solanezumab attaches to soluble amyloid and has a vascular clearance. With a trial end date in 2022, a successful outcome approval cycle would probably put market availability at about 2024, or over 20 years after the laboratory start.

Bruce's comments: *This trial is a step in the right direction. The goal is to delay progression and hope for prevention. Participants are selected with a new PET scan tracer that attaches to amyloid. Participants with amyloid are AB-positive; those without are AB-negative. Will 240 weeks be enough time to prove efficacy of an uncertain decline rate in a presymptomatic stage? Will the national goal of prevention and/or effective treatment of AD by 2025 politically influence this outcome? How will volunteers handle the knowledge of learning the possibility that AD may be in their future? Will the improved cognitive methods to measure incremental progression be deemed reliable?*

In addition to the three types of clinical trials discussed above, Alzheimer's disease neuroimaging initiative (ADNI) started in March 2005 as a three-year clinical trial using MRIs, PET Scans, and CSF to measure changes in volunteers with MCI, early AD, and normal candidates. This brilliant concept (ADNI) began a registry of people who were considered future candidates based on genetic and biomarker risk factors during qualification. A decade later, this has proven to be extremely valuable data.

The Australian Imaging, Biomarkers, and Lifestyle Flagship Study of Aging (AIBL), like ADNI, is a longitudinal biomarker cohort study that started in 2006.

Summary

In 2001, Mild Cognitive Impairment (MCI) was not recognized as a stage of AD, and those patients were not accepted for Clinical Trials. Pharmaceutical companies had high optimistic expectations of hitting that big home run. Trials were designed with criteria for accepting volunteers with disease symptoms and test scores to indicate sufficient decline from which to measure improvement.

Many failed trials were shotgun blasts at Beta Amyloid with hope that something might hit. These included vitamins, herbs, and drugs previously approved for other diseases—all without good scientific support regarding AD. The major drug candidates included vaccines and monoclonal antibodies that would eliminate plaque and/or balance the beta amyloid peptide.

A *Las Vegas Review Journal* interview with Jeffrey L. Cummings, MD, ScD on his publication [Ref. 27] highlighted fundamentals contributing to the decade of failure. Dr. Cummings stated that people were too diminished by the disease when they were given drugs to attack beta amyloid. Dr. Cummings indicated that research is too targeted and that basic research into the biology of the disease is far too low. Evidence indicates that the volunteers receiving a trial drug had already lost too many neurons for the drug to make any difference. Bruce believes that in addition to Dr. Cummings comments, increased research efforts are needed in the field of genetics, biomarkers, mitochondria, and the brain's immune system.

The key to the future is the need for a biological biomarker that can provide certainty of minute change. As of 2017, such a biomarker is still elusive, though many concepts are being pursued. Some promising biomarker candidates are (a) PET scan tracers, (b) improvements in MRI analysis, and (c) the results of the A4 trial.

Only accepting volunteers with mild or moderate disease was a misguided methodology. This was a population with MMSE scores of 15 to 26. In this range, four possibilities contributed to failed measurements. First, establishing a baseline from which to measure result was dependent upon the volunteers and such variables as the volunteers' mood, attitude, and disposition on the day of measurement. Second, disease change during these stages is uncertain and probably different for each volunteer—another variable. Third, some volunteers (like Ethel who was stable with an MMSE score of 30 for three or four years) have no change while others may have significant change—an additional variable. Fourth, volunteers with low MMSE scores (moderate range) had too much unrecoverable neuron damage to receive any benefits. Perhaps trial failures confirmed that even with large numbers of volunteers, these variables produce too many uncertainties.

Were designs of early twenty-first AD clinical trials unintentionally flawed? Was this due to the clinical trials' inclusion criteria of mild and moderate candidates? Were too many neurons lost at the Mild Stage for improvement (Ref. 16 & 39). In addition, trial end-points looked for improvement in scores from broad subjective measurement tools such as Mini-Mental State Examination (MMSE).

If current (2017) design criteria for Alzheimer's trials only accept volunteers who are classified with mild cognitive impairment (MCI) or mild AD is it realistic to continue taking medications past the mild stage of the disease? If pharmaceutical companies believed benefits are not measurable for efficacy past the mild stage, then why should patients waste money on any drugs once they are past the mild stage? What is the point if Namenda at $10/day is only a benefit for the pharmaceutical company rather than the patient?

Advances in technology, genetics, and cell biology are encouraging and have shed more light on the complexity of the challenges that researchers face. Was another trial flaw in the measuring tools used to determine change? Though the tests were the best available, they were and still are subjective assessments. Such assessments include uncertainties. Mathematics and statistics may apply justifications to minimize these uncertainties. However, if this is acceptable reasoning, then the same rational justification should apply to the creation of a signature profile to be used as a placebo signature, thereby having all patients receiving the drug.

Unknown and unresolved issues (such as pathway decline process, the neuro-immune system role, clearance system, genomic influence, sequencing, ApoE4 risks, a dependable noninvasive biomarker, improved animal models, and the interaction between beta amyloid and tau) are all career paths for future researchers. The cold, hard facts are that until the scientists gain more knowledge leading to a cure, prevention, or delay makes sense to buy time.

Buying time works for Bruce. We all need more education. In chapter 5, "The Brain," Bruce shares what he has learned about this complex human organ.

5

The Brain

Since entering the twenty-first century, information, attention, and concerns of neurological impact on the brain have heightened, with Alzheimer's disease (AD), NFL football concussions, and boxing injuries growing at an uncontrolled pace with no cure in sight. The general population has little knowledge about the most important and complex organ in the human body—the brain.

Without a cure for AD, advocates recommend caregivers and families gain as much knowledge of the disease as possible. Knowledge provides families and caregivers the ability to anticipate changes and to have intelligent discussions with doctors as the disease progresses and the patient's mental state declines. Gaining knowledge of the brain's evolution, major segments, cell types, various functions, neuron structure, and communication methodologies will increase a caregiver's capability to understand current research and assess realistic expectations. The brain is not only very complex, but it is very difficult to explain in simple terms that communicate to a nonprofessional. Bruce has chosen to tackle this task.

Overview

The brain is the control center for everything that the human body does. It contains an estimated one hundred billion neurons (nerve cells). Each neuron contains upwards of one billion parts. A very complex communication system with over a trillion connections exists in the white and grey matter of the brain where the key communication pathway unit is an *axon*. The communication system is electro-chemical, which uses a potential difference of chemical ions to transport electrical signals. The neuron structure has two major components, the nucleus and the external nucleus parts (consisting of axon, dendrites, and synapse connections). The nucleus is the central processor and the genetic storehouse. The brain also contains glial cells that perform immune system maintenance and support functions *(more later)*.

The brain is an integral part of the body, with dependency on and regulative control of the heart and lungs. Contrary to the body's ability to regenerate cells, the number of neurons in the brain is fixed for life at human birth. The brain has a separate immune system, its own maintenance system, its pain-free aspect, its cerebrospinal fluid, etc. Like the body, the brain is an evolutionary organ that has progressed and developed over millions of years.

The magnitude of parts and functions create the brain's complexity. It has the task of operating our human body from conception to death. Anomalies in any part of the brain and its functions cause abnormalities (diseases, paralysis, mutations, etc.) experienced by the brain and/or body throughout life. Such anomalies affect individual human traits, values, skills, and life paths. These anomalies become more understandable when viewed with some knowledge of this magnificent organ—the brain.

How Do We Start?

Lateral View of the Brain

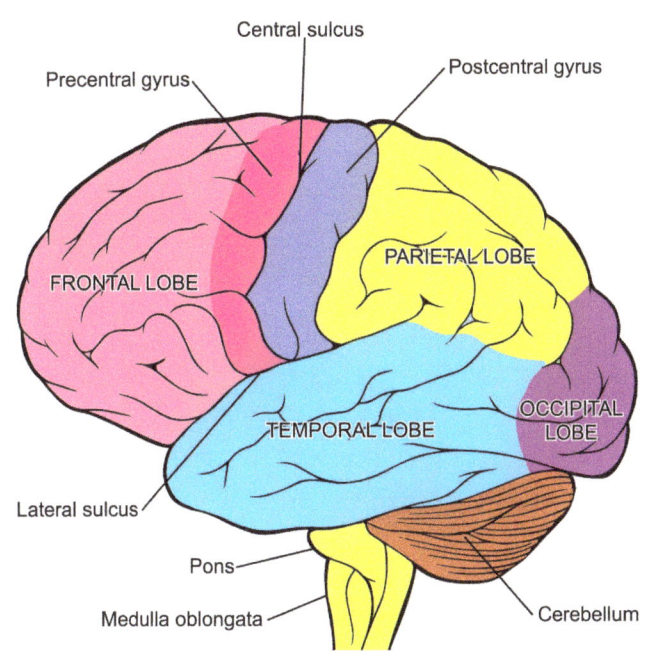

Fig. 5.1. Brain Lobes.

Figure 5.1 (showing the lobes) is one of many ways to show structural segments of the brain. As a reference overview of major segments, figure 5.1 also shows ridges and valleys. A ridge is *sulcus*. A valley is *gyrus*—the section between two ridges. The *medulla oblongata* (at the bottom) is part of an evolutionary process called the brain stem and connects to the spinal cord. The brain stem is the oldest segment of the brain. Conditions like dementia (AD, Parkinson's, Lewy body dementia, vascular disease, and frontotemporal dementia) first impact lobe areas before they reach the brain stem.

Often, the brain is discussed in two hemispheres (figure 5.2): right brain and left brain, along with white matter and grey matter. Axons reside in white matter. They form communication pathways between neurons and continue to be a major focus of AD research. Grey matter contains neurons and glial cells. The right and left hemispheres control the functions on the opposite sides of the body—right brain for left body side and left brain for right body side. The white cylinder shown between the two hemispheres in figure 5.2 depicts approximately three hundred million axons that form pathways between the two hemispheres. These are pathways that coordinate and synchronize the body's actions such as playing the piano, hitting a baseball, playing the drums, hitting a golf ball, etc.

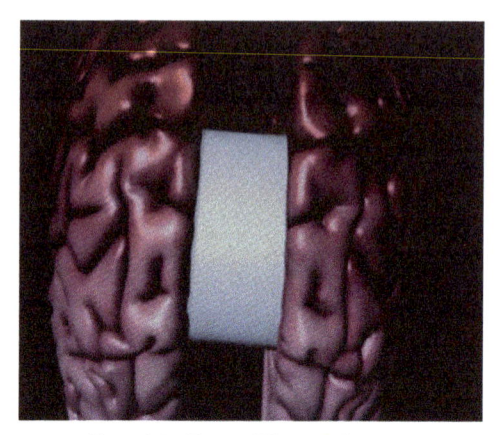

Fig. 5.2. Brain Hemispheres.

Norden, Jeanette, Vanderbilt University, Nashville, TN "Lecture Central Nervous System—Subdivisions," Understanding the Brain, The Great Course, 2007, DVD

Glial cells form a protective sheath around axons, along with acting like a trash collector for toxins identified by the immune system. The roles of glial cells are better appreciated as research discovers new functions that they are performing. Glial cells and the immune system are areas for additional research as they are far from being well understood.

The book, *Super Brain*, by Deepak Chopra and Rudolph E. Tanzi (2012) described the evolution of the brain in three stages: the reptilian which controls vital functions, the limbic which records memories and emotions, and the neocortex which governs executive functions and learning abilities (figure 5.3). From an AD viewpoint, it appears to be last in, segment or brain stem evolved first, along with spinal cord neurons. The brain stem contains the instinctive elements for living and survival. Most of these essentials are functions that we take for granted such as breathing, temperature regulation, body organ control, the senses (taste, sight, touch, smell, hearing), walking, running, eating, elimination, reproduction, and others. Representatives of this stage were probably among the earliest humans.

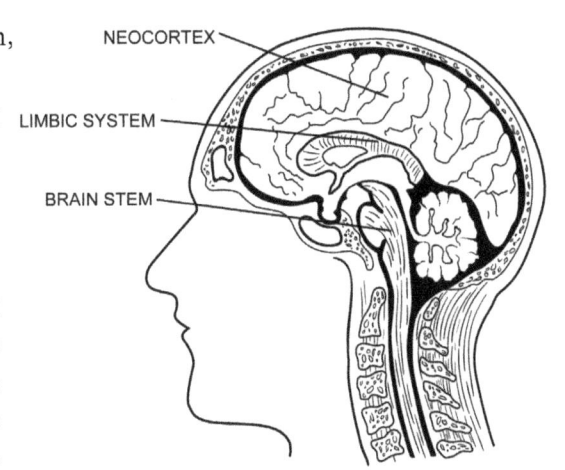

Fig. 5.3. Brain Evolution.

Who was the first man and how did he develop? Eugène Dubois, a Dutch surgeon, found the remains of the first *Homo erectus* individual (*Trinil 2*) in Indonesia in 1891. In 1894, Dubois named the species *Pithecanthropus erectus,* or *erect Ape-man*. At that time, *Pithecanthropus* (later changed to *Homo erectus*) was the most primitive and smallest-brained of all known early human species.

Homo erectus (meaning upright man) lived around 1.9 million years ago, based on the earliest fossil evidence, and extending to around 75,000 years ago. How would a *Homo erectus* brain compare to what we know about the brain of today? How did the brain evolve from that period to today? Based on the behavioral patterns of evolution theory, is it reasonable to assume that a *Homo erectus* brain may have been just the basic stem portion of a modern brain?

The limbic system presumably evolved next, adding language and emotions. Language occurred after the body developed the larynx bone structure. Emotions such as love, desire, fear, and pride advanced humans. Representatives of this period probably included the people in the Stone, Bronze, and Iron ages (period of 200,000 to 10,000 years ago), before the first recording of human history.

These people migrated to form different races and cultures. They developed lasting relationships and created communities of families. The neocortex brain region added the executive functions of intellect, thinking, reasoning, and decision making. Emotional controls, creative thinking, and the power to choose values, either good or bad, became part of a human with the addition of the neocortex. Is the brain still evolving?

Homo sapiens (wise man), including Neanderthals, are considered the earliest species of modern man. From 200,000 years to the present, the modern brain appears to have made significant development and growth along with body development. How did this occur? Did the brain evolve from the brain stem to adding the limbic system and then adding the neocortex, or were all today's one hundred billion neurons there in both *Homo erectus* and *Homo sapiens*—with unconnected pathways? Human recorded history is less than 10,000 years old, so anyone's opinion may be as good as anyone else's. The opinion presented here is that not only has evolution brought us to where we are today but that the brain is still evolving and will continue to evolve into the future, if not delayed or destroyed by natural laws or overpopulation. Learning how the brain develops and matures, along with its functions, provides a tremendous advantage for dealing with life's challenges in a positive and satisfying way.

Who is to say what is next for future generations? Today's focus should be on the present and how individuals deal with life in the societal, political, technological, and environmental period in which they live. Those of us who are part of the "lucky few generation" (described by Elwood D. Carlson, Ph.D. in his 2008 book titled, *The Lucky Few: Between the Greatest Generation and the Baby Boom*) should be very appreciative of the period in which they lived. I am.

Brain Development

Most men probably take their partner's nine-month pregnancy as just a normal event without knowledge of the complex events that occur during that time and shortly thereafter. Understanding the brain development sheds light on the magnificent process that produces a normal human birth. The following intends to give an appreciation of the important pregnancy cycle that many of us take for granted in our culture and society. During the first month of pregnancy, a neural plate (Figure 5.4) is formed in eighteen days. The neural plate cells proliferate at the edges, folding up to form the neural tube (Figure 5.5) by four weeks. The portion above the tube in Figure 5.5 becomes skin.

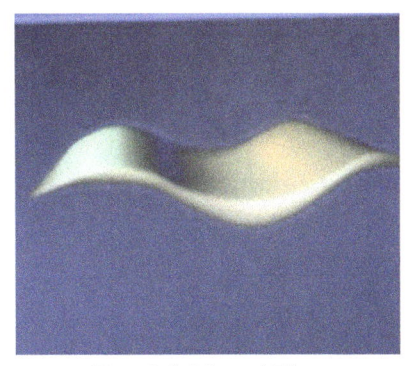

Fig. 5.4. Neural Plate.

Norden, Jeanette, Vanderbilt University, Nashville, TN "Lecture Central Nervous System—Development," Understanding the Brain, The Great Course, 2007, DVD

The tube begins the central nervous system (CNS) consisting of the brain and spinal cord. Figure 5.5 shows the formation of the brain's ventricular system in the central cavity that becomes the interface with the spinal cord and the passage of *cerebrospinal fluid* (CSF).

Weeks 12 through 20 become a critical period (defined as the start and finish of an event that must occur for a normal birth) during which the neurons (Figure 5.7) and glial cells are generated from progenitor cells. Progenitor cells are like stem cells that can divide and duplicate. One hundred billion neurons, along with up to five times as many glial cells, are generated during this time. Progenitor cells are limited to this period for duplication. At completion of the process, glial cells remove the progenitor cells from the brain. Glial cells guide the neu-

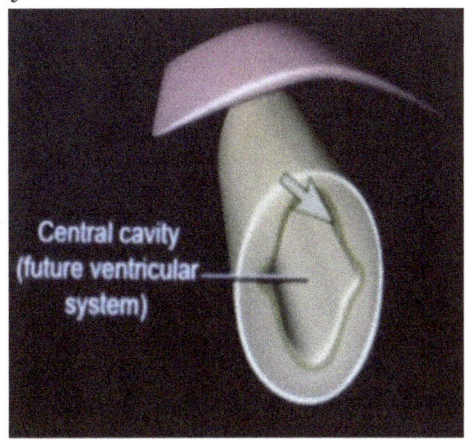

Fig. 5.5. Neural Tube.

Norden, Jeanette, Vanderbilt University, Nashville, TN "Lecture Central Nervous System—Development," Understanding the Brain, The Great Course, 2007, DVD

rons to their location. Grey matter develops along with the neurons. Axons and dendrites (*more later*) develop along with white matter to form the communication structure and network—the nervous system. Neurons are in the spinal cord and the eyes. Glial cells are like stem cells that divide to replace cells that die. Neurons do not divide.

Third Trimester to Age Two Years

Figure 5.6 shows the brain shape from four weeks to birth. The connection of the dendrite and axons begin to materialize during the final trimester and continue through two years of age to complete basic functions. Prior to birth, there is a reduction of neurons as the brain eliminates any unneeded neurons used during the development process. With the advancement in medicine today, freezing and storing a newborn's umbilical cord in a medical bank for potential future use might be a consideration. However, biotechnology and genetics could make this unnecessary.

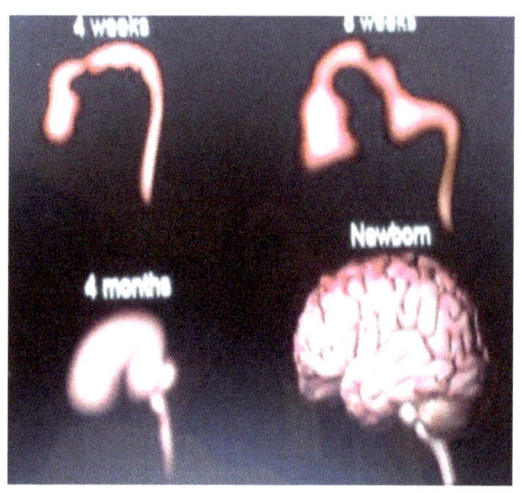

Figure 5.6. Brain Development.

Norden, Jeanette, Vanderbilt University, Nashville, TN "Lecture Central Nervous System—Development," Understanding the Brain, The Great Course, 2007, DVD

The significance of proper care of the mother's lifestyle during pregnancy is critical to the development, birth, and growth of a newborn. Studies of children in Africa and India show the lack of development both physically and mentally are due to lack of proper nutrients from the mother during development period and the first two years of life. Think about how a mother on drugs might affect the development of the fetus.

Axon and dendrite connections continue to evolve throughout life, but the needed pathways are developed from the third trimester to two years. A child learns as these pathways are connected. Though a child cannot initially talk, its sensory inputs and memory storage are functioning. Therefore, parents should consider taking advantage of this capability. Try implanting values, words, stories and math during pregnancy and at an early age. You can even tell the unborn fetus as well as the child that you love them now and always.

At birth, the child has all the neurons it will ever have. The glial cells are different as they can divide and replicate throughout life. To date, approximately 150 different neuron types have been identified, but there are only two types of glial cells—microglia and macroglia. (*See section on glial cells, later.*)

Neuron

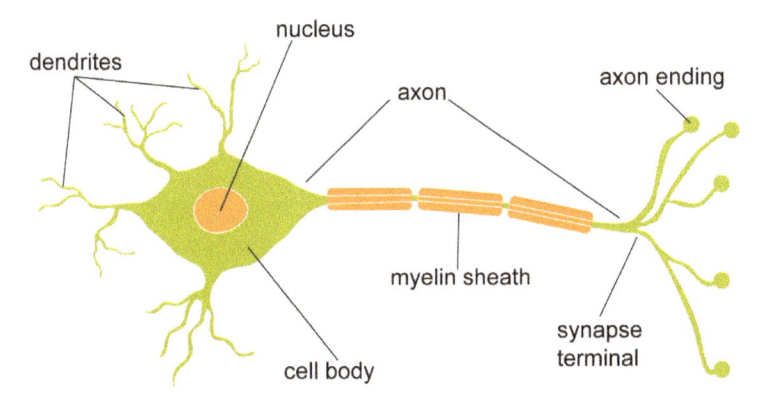

Fig. 5.7. Neuron.

Figure 5.7 shows a neuron. The axon, dendrites, myelin sheath, axon endings, and synapses are described below. These are the external parts of a neuron. The nucleus contains internal parts where chromosomes, DNA, genes, RNA, proteins, amino acids, and sequencing, control and process the functions of the human body through electrical and chemical mechanisms. Chemicals such as hydrogen, oxygen, potassium, phosphorous, sodium, carbon, and many others are obtained through diet, thereby creating a chemical factory of elements operating the magnificent system that is our human body.

The neuron has an internal and external structure. The internal cell (nucleus) is the control center for the body. The nucleus is composed of chromosomes, genes, and DNA (genetic material) that processes instructions to control the body (more on the nucleus later). The external cell is composed of the axon, dendrite, and synapse. Alzheimer's research and clinical trials focused on a hypothesis that amyloid plaque has accumulated in this external area and eventually leads to the death of neurons. After two decades of research and clinical trials, the hypothesis is not yet proven. Could it be that the neurons do not die, but just the pathways are destroyed? (Unlikely, but…) Therefore, could technology in the future create new connections to restore neuron pathways and memory? (Food for thought.)

Axons

The axon is like an electric wire with a myelin sheath (insulation) around it. The axon's myelin sheath is formed by astrocytes (the most abundant glial cells). Axons are nerve fibers, formed in sections, which establish part of the brain's communication pathways. The sections allow axon branches to develop as needed. There are long and short axons. Short axons are for neurons within nuclei (group of neurons) or closed nuclei like in the cerebellum, where over 50 percent of the total neurons are found. There are three types of long axon pathways. The first is the association pathway within each hemisphere that connects paths of the cortex. The second pathway is the commissural that connects across the hemispheres (*see white section in Figure 5.2*). There is a bundle of three hundred million axon cross-connections to the opposite hemisphere. The third is the projection pathway that makes direct connections between neurons in different parts of the brain along with connections to the spinal cord and body. An example of a long axon is like a motor pathway that goes from the brain to the spinal cord to control body limbs. Microscope evaluation of these axons identified them as white. Therefore, axons reside in the brain's white matter. Neurons do not replicate, but axons can form new pathways. Therefore, assuming the neuron does not die, but the communication chain is lost by a destroyed axon or dendrite, could it then be possible to create a bypass, like a heart bypass? Could there be reserve neurons? So far, as of 2017, there are no answers to these questions.

Dendrites and Axon Hillock

Dendrites are like the branches of a tree. They have spines (like twigs of a branch). They function as the receiving element for the neuron cell body. Dendrites have different shapes and branch formations, like trees. Dendrites are shaped differently for each type of neuron—150 types have been identified to date. Figure 5.8 shows a representative number of dendrites. Each spoke (branch) has spines (twigs) and receptors to receive information from other neurons. Depending on the function defined by the nucleus, the number of dendrites can be a few or possibly in the hundreds. The axon hillock shown in Figure 5.8 provides an interface between the cell body (nucleus) and the axon. Its function is to determine what level and type of electro-chemical signal will be released down the axon.

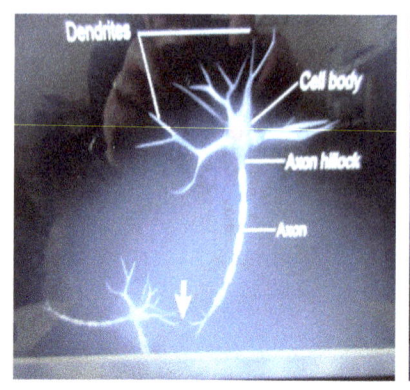

Fig. 5.8. Representative Neuron.

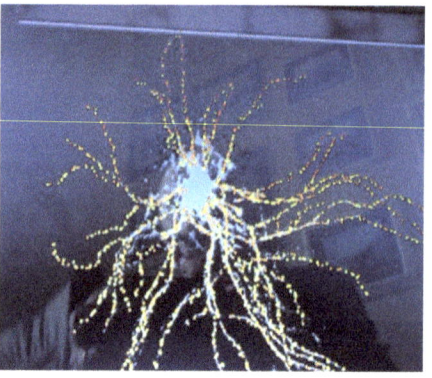

Fig. 5.9. Many Dendrites.

Norden, Jeanette, Vanderbilt University, Nashville, TN "Lecture Central Nervous System—Cellular Organization," Understanding the Brain, The Great Courses, 2007, DVD

Norden, Jeanette, Vanderbilt University, Nashville, TN "Lecture Central Nervous System—Cellular Organization," Understanding the Brain, The Great Courses, 2007, DVD

Figure 5.9 shows a neuron with many dendrite spines. Each dot is a synapse. There are one hundred billion neurons in the brain and an estimated one hundred trillion synapses. This provides an appreciation of what researchers face in just the external portion of a neuron in trying to find a cause and cure for Alzheimer's and other brain diseases. It becomes more overwhelming when the nucleus is included.

Communication

Neuron communication with each other and with the body is amazing, technical, and complex. The external cell communication key elements include the axon hillock, axons, dendrites, synapses, and neurotransmitters. Then there are electro-chemical signals that excite and/or inhibit the release of neurotransmitters into extra cellular space. The arrow in figure 5.8 is pointing to the area between the axon terminal and a connecting dendrite spine. This area is a *synapse*.

The axon hillock triggers an electro-chemical signal that travels down the axon to the *presynaptic axon terminal* for chemical processing. Figure 5.10 shows the presynaptic and postsynaptic dendrite spine terminals. The *synaptic vesicle* contains neurotransmitters of which there are sixty known types to date. Glutamate and gamma amino butyric acid (GABA) are neuro-transmitters (chemical messengers).

Glutamate is an excitatory neurotransmitter, while GABA mainly causes an inhibitory action. Other neurotransmitters include dopamine, norepinephrine, serotonin, acetylcholine, and many others. When an electro-chemical signal (a positive or negatively charged atom) from the axon hillock reaches the presynaptic area terminal, a cascade of events starts. A receptor on the terminal's membrane opens whereby a calcium ion from extracellular space enters the terminal and triggers the release of neurotransmitters from the synaptic vesicle. These chemicals locate matching membrane positions for their release (see little red dots in fig. 5.10) into the synapse area. These neurotransmitters then search for matching receptors on the postsynaptic dendrite spine terminal to convey the message to the dendrite spine of the receiving neuron. The presynaptic area terminal opens a receptor for reuptake (arrow in figure 10) of excess neurotransmitters and repackages them for future use. Other neurotransmitters, remaining in extracellular space, are gathered up by microglia cells. The postsynaptic area is a prime spot for plaque accumulation in AD. In addictive diseases (drugs or alcohol) the reuptake receptor becomes damaged leaving excess neurotransmit-

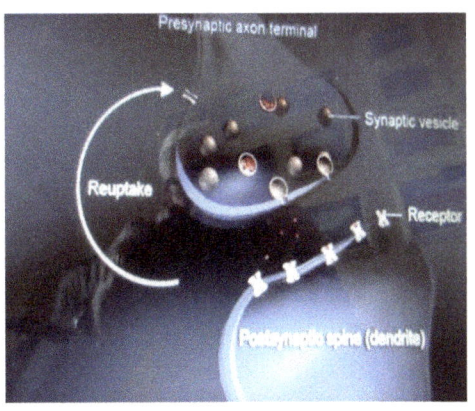

Fig. 5.10. Synapse.

Norden, Jeanette, Vanderbilt University, Nashville, TN "Lecture Central Nervous System—Cellular Organization" Understanding the Brain, The Great Course, 2007, DVD

ters (such as dopamine) to provide more input to the postsynaptic receptors, thereby creating an ever-changing normal demand level for the function (drinking alcohol).

Cell Nucleus

The nucleus of a cell is like an Intel chip in a cell phone. It is the central processor of the brain and body. A nucleus contains more than one billion subparts and is 70 percent water. The internal cell contains a person's individual makeup of chromosomes, genes, and DNA (along with other elements) which guide the interaction between neurons to achieve the behavior functions of a human. The external portion of the cell discussed above performs many duties like a computer server/router in a large computer system where it receives inputs and routes the information to where it goes for display, print, storage, or further transmission to other parts of the system. This is like your eyes sending information to stop moving your hand to the burner on the stove because it is on and will burn you. The number of neurons that are involved is uncertain but probably millions of neurons participate in less than a second.

As functional actions and behaviors are discussed later, reference to the above will provide an appreciation of the complexity of action by the brain required to accomplish processes that we do not even realize—until those processes do not work.

Glial Cells

Glial cells are found in both grey and white matter. Glial cell research is an area of opportunity for any researcher. Knowledge gains of glial involvement is producing continued discoveries.

There are two classes of glial cells: microglia and macroglia. *Microglia* role is keeping the brain in a homeostatic (balanced) condition. This is performed in many ways such as providing antigens (like immune T-cells in the body) from the brain's immune system when an anomaly occurs or performing housecleaning duties. They gather and take care of waste (dead neurons, demyelinated axons, toxic proteins, etc.) from the brain and processed by way of the spinal cord to the body's elimination system. There are three types of *macroglia* cells: the oligodendrocyte (o-lig-o-den-dro-cyte), the astrocytes, and Schwann cells.

Oligodendrocytes form the myelin sheath that wraps around the axon. These same cells form part of the blood brain barrier (BBB) by tightly wrapping around the blood vessels and act as a filter for the transport of nutrients and chemicals allowed from the blood to the neurons. Medical drugs must factor this barrier into their design. This has been a major problem in Alzheimer's research, whereby drugs for preventing fibrils and tangles in the tau protein have had problems penetrating the BBB—thus far. A new hypothesis is that amyloid plaque in AD attacks the myelin protection, destroying the associated pathway.

Astrocytes have many roles. Their initial function begins in the womb, guiding neurons to their locations in the brain. (This is like an automatic mail sorting system where letters are like neurons and get off at the right zip code). The area between neurons in the brain is extracellular space. This space contains charged atoms with ions such as potassium, calcium, chloride, etc. which are regulated by the astrocyte cells. The astrocytes also act as the protector for neurons. When a toxic substance is detected, the astrocytes surround the substance, forming a scar-like covering. Unfortunately, multiple sclerosis (multiple scars), an autoimmune disease, causes the immune system to send astrocytes to attack healthy cells, which creates a scar and causes the death of the neuron. This leads to disability as communication pathways break down.

Schwann cells are involved in many important aspects of peripheral nerve biology such as the conduction of nervous impulses along axons, nerve developments and regeneration as well as trophic support for neurons, etc.

Genetics

What are genetics? What is a genome? What are chromosomes, genes, gene sequencing, proteins, and amino acids? How do they all work together? What impact do these have on our health and disease? In brief, all of them are the magnificent parts of a beautiful organ—*the brain*.

Relative to the brain, *genetics* is a study of the parts of the nucleus of a neuron (figure 5.7) that control and regulate activity in the brain as well as the evolution of these parts through their sex cells and non-sex cells inheritance of chromosomes, genes, and DNA. In addition, genetics includes the study of the transfer of genetic material to define the amino acids for proteins.

Chromosomes

Chromosomes are the starting point. Most humans have forty-six chromosomes. There are twenty-two pairs, one set from each parent (=44). Paired chromosomes are *autosomes*. The embryo receives X default sex chromosomes from the female parent, and either X or Y sex chromosomes from a male parent. Gender is determined by whether the sperm provides either an X or Y sex chromosome. Millions of sperm cells search to find and fertilize the egg.

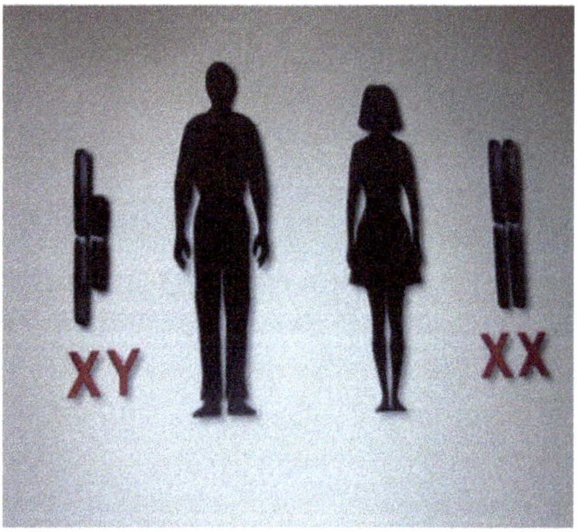

Fig. 5.11. Chromosomes.

David Savada PhD, *Pritzker Family Foundation Professor of Biology, Claremont Colleges*, "Lecture Genes and Chromosomes," *Understanding Genetics*, The Great Courses. 2008 DVD

Each sperm cell carries different generational combinations of DNA. A storehouse of eggs, that also has generational combinations of DNA, ovulates one. The various combinations of these DNA are an evolutionary mixture passed down through generations. The one-in-a-million sperm cell's DNA that fertilizes the ovulated egg creates the unique characteristics and inherited traits in the embryo. This is consistent with Darwin's theory of natural selection and why traits of our parents, grandparents, great-grandparents, etc. become recognizable.

So, what happens if we get either X or Y from the male parent? The embryo development starts without gender recognition and proceeds on a default mode of X. During embryo development, if the sperm provided a Y chromosome, a gene called *sex determining region Y (SRY)* signals for a gonad hormone to create testosterone, thus creating a male. If the sperm provides an X chromosome, the default mode continues and signals for the gonad hormone to proceed to create estrogen, thus creating a female.

Abnormalities can occur in cell division during embryogenesis that result in either X, XXY, or XXXY. Thus, if the sperm provides both X and Y, one would be recessive—not dominant, therefore inactive. If the Y chromosome were inactive, it would be unable to generate the SRY gene on the Y chromosomes, thereby leaving a female with an inactive Y chromosome—likewise for a second X in males. Could such abnormalities be an influence of gender preference later in. life? The Y chromosome of the male is smaller and has fewer genes than the female X chromosomes.

Chromosomes provide a backbone to which genes are attached. This backbone is a sugar-phosphate substance, deoxyribonucleic acid (DNA) that was discovered in the first half of the twentieth century. Identifying genes on chromosomes is an ongoing activity in genetic research today. A more difficult ongoing research is identifying the functions associated with each chromosome.

Early onset of Alzheimer's disease (about age thirty-five) has two genes identified as risk factors. These genes are presenilin-1 that is located on chromosome 14 and presenilin-2 located on chromosome 1. Late onset Alzheimer's disease (symptoms begin showing at age sixty-five and over) has identified apolipoprotein E gene as a risk factor due to a dominant E4 allele that is located on chromosome 19. Alleles are alternative forms of the same gene, received either from a parent or by a mutation.

Genes

Genes are the brain's microchips. The nervous system operates remarkably with an estimated 26,000 genes. Comparatively, rice (a grain) has over 35,000 genes. Genes contain a genetic code (discussed later) as well as the ability to synthesize proteins (discussed later). DNA provides the brain a virtual reality capability and operates from a coding mechanism that controls and regulates the brain's signals to and from senses, organs, and limbs. DNA uses a messenger called mRNA to provide instructions for creating proteins (more later).

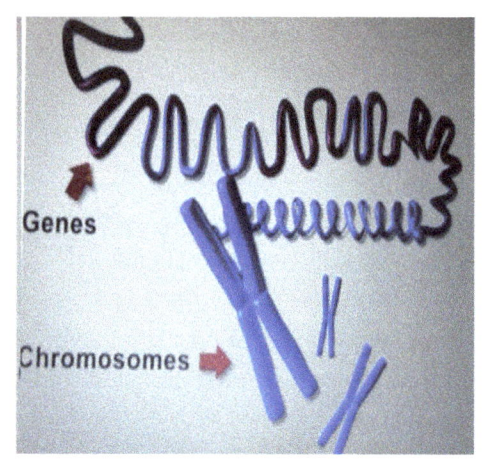

Fig. 5.12. Chromosomes & Genes.

David Savada PhD, *Pritzker Family Professor of Biology, Claremont Colleges*, "Lecture Genes and Chromosomes," *Understanding Genetics*, The Great Courses. 2008 DVD

The estimated 26,000 genes contained in each cell are allotted across twenty-two pairs of chromosomes. Each gene has a specific order and location on one of forty-four chromosomes. Each parent provides one copy of a gene in the same order and location on a specific chromosome, thus creating the twenty-two pairs of *autosomes* (nonsex chromosomes). Each autosome has two copies of the same gene at the same location (figure 5.12). The autosomes' copies are distinguished by their genotype (genetic makeup—DNA) and their phenotype function (appearance, traits, and characteristics). The two copies of autosome genes are called *alleles*—ApoE3 and ApoE4. Chromosomes vary in the number of genes they contain based on function. Some chromosomes contain millions of genes—multiples of many genes.

The brain and human body function through genetic material (DNA) along with RNA, proteins, and *mitochondria DNA*. Mitochondria are double *membranes organelles (subpart of a cell)* that provide chemical energy, needed by a cell.

A membrane is a boundary or enclosure (like a bottle, fence, wall, etc.). A membrane also encloses the nucleus of the cell. Mitochondria has its own DNA makeup (different than autosomes)

Genes mutate. A mutation is a permanent change to a gene. A new mutated gene passes to the next generation (evolution). Gene mutation can be from the environment, behavior, disease, or error in replication. Genetics and Genes are complicated subjects with many subparts that play vital roles in the normal and abnormal functions of the brain and human body.

Other parts within a cell nucleus include proteins, messenger RNAs (mRNA), amino acids, hormones, a genetic code, polymers, monomers, nucleotides, and sequencing—overwhelming! With additional information, these challenging terms become comprehensible.

Understandably, we trust our medical professionals to take care of us—and rightfully so. However, being knowledgeable helps us guide our personal medical decisions. An overview into the genetic content of genes through their genetic material (DNA, RNA, and proteins) follows.

Deoxyribonucleic Acid (DNA)

In 1944, Oswald Avery, together with colleagues Colin MacLeod and Maclyn McCarty, published a landmark paper on the transforming ability of DNA. This opened the door for genetics and the biotechnology industry that followed. Despite this historic discovery and publication, Avery and colleagues were not awarded a Nobel Prize. Deoxyribonucleic Acid (DNA) is a molecule (an electrically neutral group of two or more atoms held together by chemical bonds). It carries genetic information used in the development, functioning, and reproduction of all known living organisms.

During the first twenty weeks of gestation, genes are placed along the backbone in a specific order on a specific chromosome, thereby establishing a specific location for each gene. This results in long fibrous strands of DNA (one from the mother and one from the father) that become genetic material called *polymers* (figure 5.13).

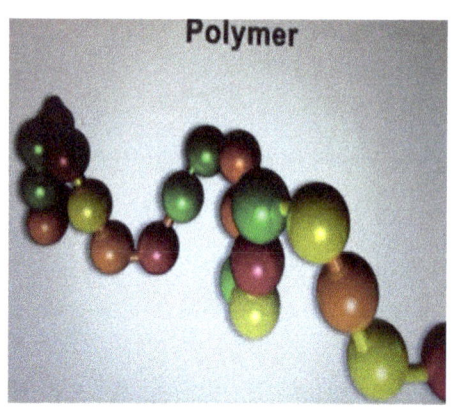

Fig. 5.13. Polymers.

David Savada PhD, *Pritzker Family Foundation Professor of Biology, Claremont Colleges*, "Lecture *DNA Structure and Replication*" *Understanding Genetics,* The Great Courses. 2008 DVD

Think of a *polymer* as a long chain and *monomers* as four distinct types of charms hanging repeatedly on the chain. The monomers are *nucleotides* (chemical compounds). The four nucleotides are *adenine (A), guanine (G), thymine (T)* and *cytosine (C) (*figure 5.14). The nucleotides' names are seldom used, but A, T, G, C are extremely important as these are the keys to DNA. Nucleotide A is always paired with T, and G is always paired with C (A=T and G=C). If the nucleotide (monomer) from the mother is A, then it will always be paired with the T nucleotide on the father's fibrous strand forming a pair. The same applies for G and C. Each gene varies in the number of nucleotide pairs in accordance with the function of the gene. These pairs within genes range from hundreds up to millions. This is part of the complexity facing researchers.

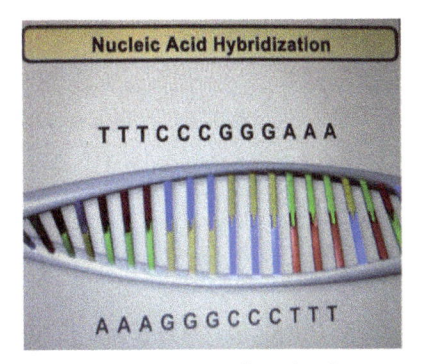

Fig. 5.15. Nucleic Acid Hybridization.

David Savada PhD, *Pritzker Family Foundation Professor of Biology, Claremont Colleges*, "Lecture DNA Structure and Replication" *Understanding Genetics,* The Great Courses. 2008 DVD

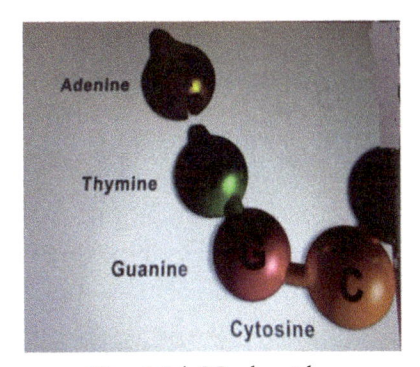

Fig. 5.14. Nucleotides.

David Savada PhD, *Pritzker Family Foundation Professor of Biology, Claremont Colleges*, "Lecture DNA Structure and Replication" *Understanding Genetics,* The Great Courses. 2008 DVD

Example: Mother's Nucleotide Strand = ACGTTGACAATTGCCG
Father's Nucleotide Strand = TGCAACTG TTAACGGC

This combination of nucleotide pairs is called *nucleic acid hybridization* (figure 5.15). Each letter represents a chemical compound. The gene considers this chemical data as information to be used to process or receive instructions associated with its functions. For example, an insulin gene has 493 nucleotide pairs. Other genes vary in pairs up to the millions, with upward of 26,000 genes and varied numbers up to millions of nucleotides and various combination possibilities. Finding the one nucleotide pair causing a medical problem is indicative of complexity.

In 1953, James Watson and Francis Crick concluded that the DNA molecule consists of two biopolymer strands (A=T and/or G=C) coiled around each other and only fit perfectly as a double helix of polymers (figure 5.16). In addition, Alfred Hershey and Martha Chase performed tests that proved *DNA was genetic material.* As late twentieth and early twenty-first century discoveries, DNA and its sequencing provided tremendous advances and hope for the future. However, genetics is still in its infancy due to the magnitude and complexities associated with the varied combination of nucleotide pairs involved as well as other issues (such as lack of identification of the functions of all chromosomes and genes). What a wonderful opportunity for a bright young student!

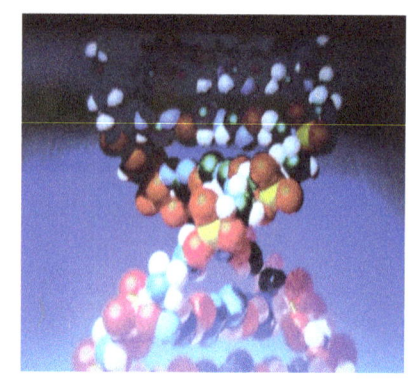

Fig. 5.16. Polymer Double Helix.

David Savada PhD, *Pritzker Family Foundation Professor of Biology, Claremont Colleges,* "Lecture *DNA Structure and Replication*" *Understanding Genetics,* The Great Courses. 2008 DVD

Figure 5.17 summarizes genetic material. The green color represents deoxyribonucleic acid (DNA), which contains chromosomes, genes, and nucleotides.

| <-------------------------Chromosome--------------------------> ||||
| Gene PSEN1—ATG | Gene PSEN 2—TGC | Gene ApoE—GCA | Gene TREM2—CAT |

Figure 5.17. DNA.

There are forty-four chromosomes in twenty-two pairs containing various lengths and number of genes. The 26,000 genes are specifically located on a chromosome. Figure 5.17 shows a simple example of four genes (PSEN1, PSEN2, ApoE, and TREM2) identified as AD risk factors. Each of the letters (ATG, TGC, GCA, and CAT) represent nucleotides (basic structural units) that form sequences of nucleotides of hundreds to millions on each gene, thereby creating its genetic material. There are about 3.2 billion nucleotides in the 26,000 genes that are located on twenty-two pairs of chromosomes. This averages about 100,000 nucleotides per gene or 50,000 nucleotide base pairs. A description of *genetic material* that could take many books to define follows in very broad and simple terms.

Genetic Material

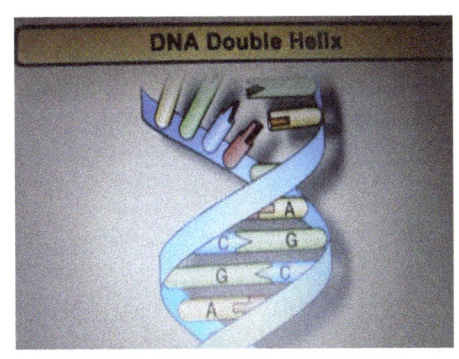

Fig. 5.18. DNA Double Helix.

David Savada PhD, *Pritzker Family Foundation Professor of Biology, Claremont Colleges*, "Lecture *DNA Structure and Replication*" *Understanding Genetics*, The Great Courses. 2008 DVD

Figure 5.18 shows the DNA double helix. The two strands of DNA, one provided by the father and one by the mother, contain genes and nucleotides that form pairs (A=T and G=C). They are loosely connected by a hydrogen atom.

The human genome (the totality of genetic material) is the complete set of nucleic acid (nucleotides) sequence for humans (homo sapiens) and encoded as DNA within the twenty-two chromosome pairs inside the cell nucleus.

The requirements for a gene's *genetic material* are (1) It has *information storage,* (2) it must *accurately duplicate helix (replication),* (3) it must be *expressed as a phenotype, and* (4) it can *change (mutate). Where is the evidence?*

The nucleotides satisfy the requirement for *information storage*. Nucleotides are like letters in the alphabet. They are paired in a DNA double helix formation (figure 5.18). As alphabet letters form words, and words form sentences to provide information, the genes' nucleotides initiate sequences that become instructions, thereby demonstrating the requirement for information storage.

Figure 5.19 shows *replication*. An enzyme begins the process by dividing the double helix into two parts, thereby splitting the nucleotide pairs, leaving one strand with an A and the other strand with a T. The process continues with the strand that has an A receiving a new T and, likewise, for the other strand where the T receives a new A and continues until the gene is replicated and a new DNA is formed. This process meets the requirement for *accurate duplication*. Errors sometimes occur, though most errors are corrected. Those not corrected are variants (mutations).

What is a *phenotype*? A phenotype is the observable properties and physical characteristics (traits) of an organism. For example, an eye is an organism with an observable property of color. The color's physical characteristics are shades of blue, green, brown, or hazel. Other examples are races, hair, skin, height, etc. DNA that is inherited from the sperm and egg influences these traits.

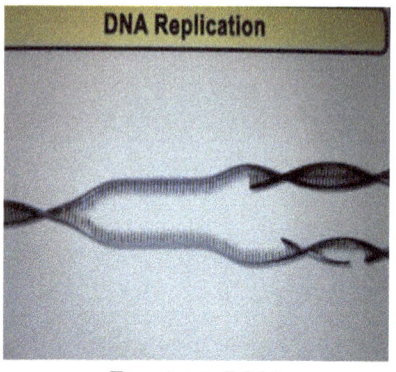

Fig. 5.19. DNA Accurate Replication.

David Savada PhD, *Pritzker Family Foundation Professor of Biology, Claremont Colleges*, "Lecture *DNA Structure and Replication*" *Understanding Genetics*, The Great Courses. 2008 DVD

What does *expressed* mean? There are two copies of each gene (one from the father's sperm and one from the mother's egg). These copies are called *alleles*. At conception, two of the four alleles are selected (how is unknown) and become a part of natural selection for determining the embryo's *genetic material*. Gene alleles are referred to as genotypes. The gene's alleles (from whatever generational combination) plus the environment (part of the world or area where you live) determine and express these phenotypes or traits. Example of the different results of the expression are the different skin colors from various parts of the world, different hair color, different features and traits in humans, thus demonstrating DNA expression as phenotype.

What is a *mutation*? Mutations occur in many ways that are extremely complex with a large variety of effects, both beneficial and negative (such as cancer). Genetic variations can be as small as a single nucleotide base-pair change (insertion or deletion) or as large as the gain or loss of multiple chromosomes. A single nucleotide base-pair change provides examples. A mutation is a permanent change in a gene's nucleotide sequence.

Nucleotide letters shown in table 5.1 represent a gene's meaningful information like alphabet letters form words (see column 4). The word example shows the effect of such a change on word meaning. A mutant sequence letter (indicated in red) changes the meaning of the gene's instruction or information (like the word example change shown in column 4). The red *!* indicates the missing nucleotide. As changing the word *plus* to *plush* would be incorrect in a sentence, a nucleotide sequence is the same. Mutations can cause disease or be beneficial and evolutionary. Mutations cause various diseases which verify that DNA can change. Thus, DNA satisfies the requirements for *genetic material*.

Table 5.1. Mutation Example.

Type of Mutation	Normal Nucleotide (N) Sequence	Mutated Nucleotide Sequence	Word Example
Replication Error Added pair	ATCG GTAC TAGC CATG	CATCG GTACA GTAGC CATGT	EACH... TEACH PLUS... PLUSH
Replication Error Missing Pair	CTTAGCTGTCA GAATCGACAGT	CTTAGC!GTCA GAATCG!CAGT	REACHING TEACHING
Reverse of Nucleotides	TCG AGC	GCT CGA	DOG GOD
Nucleotide Change	GTAC CATG	GTTC CAAG	Some Same

An unfortunate mutation example is the addition of a third copy of chromosome #22, causing Down syndrome. The amyloid precursor protein gene is on chromosome #22. Excess amyloid production is a characteristic of AD. Many Down syndrome patients experience many of AD type symptoms. Could the future hold elimination of the third #22 chromosomes by using CRISPR/Cas9? (*You be the judge after reading chapter 7.*)

With the establishment that DNA is genetic material, next is the question of how genes process instructions to organisms. Here again, the beauty and complexity of our human brain and body organs start to come into focus as we will see how this genetic material orchestrates the proteins used throughout our body. Since genetics is at its infancy, the future holds hope. The *double helix* and proof of *genetic material* were discovered in 1953. A promising revolutionary genetic tool (CRISPR/Cas9) that can change nucleotides and alleles was introduced in 2012 (*more in chapter 7*).

The Genetic Process

With genetics covered from a structural viewpoint and the confirmation of DNA as genetic material, the process of how genetic material is used to code proteins follows.

The process was only determined in the last fifty-five years. Completion of the first Human Genome Project was in 2003, with the successful sequencing of a genome, thereby determining the exact order of the base pairs in a segment of DNA. Current knowledge claims that only 2 percent of 3.2 billion nucleotides are for gene coding. Genetics will be the job opportunity of the future to determine the roles of the other 98 percent of the nucleotides.

The genetic process involves trans-lation from nucleotides to amino acids, a transformation of coded information from the location of the nucleotides to a site where protein synthesis (making proteins) takes place. A messenger RNA (mRNA) transports RNA codons to the protein site (ribosome).

To use DNA genetic material, nucleotide instructions need translation from their current chemical structure to specify a protein chemical structure—amino acids (figure 5.20). Proteins have twenty different amino acids. Nucleotides have four chemicals (letters A, T, C, and G). So, how does the human body process four nucleotide letters to specify which of twenty amino acids to use to make a protein? Like the British deciphering of the German code during World War II, genetic researchers were faced with the problem of deciphering code that cells use.

Marshall Nirenberg solved the problem in 1961 by deciphering the cells' code, which required combinations of four nucleotides to twenty specific amino acids. Therefore, Nirenberg determined that the third power of four or sixty-four (4x4x4) would provide a three-letter nucleotide combination or codon triplet that allows identification of each one of the twenty amino acids (figure 21). Using DNA transcription (the process by which the information in one strand of DNA is copied into a new molecule of messenger RNA), Nirenberg performed tests to decipher which codon triplet identified which amino acid and produced the genetic code. The next problem was to determine how the specified code was transcribed to amino acid and proteins.

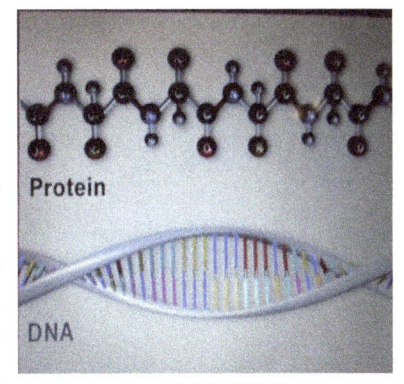

Fig. 5.20. DNA to Protein.

David Savada PhD, *Pritzker Family Foundation Professor of Biology, Claremont Colleges*, "Lecture *DNA Structure and Replication*" *Understanding Genetics,* The Great Courses. 2008 DVD

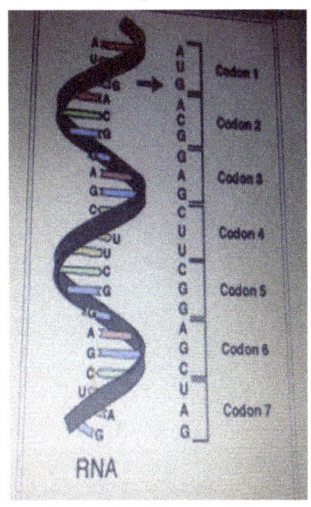

Figure 5.21. RNA Triplets.

Transcription is the first step of gene expression in which a segment of DNA is copied into ribonucleic acid (RNA) where the RNA segment is a single strand of the DNA genetic material (figure 22). RNA has many functions. One function is to analyze the DNA and create the codon's triplet instructions for defining amino acids. A second RNA function create a messenger RNA (mRNA).

The mRNA transports the codon triplet instructions to the cell's *ribosome.* Ribosomes have two subunits. The small subunit reads the RNA's codon instructed triplets and translates them into amino acids. The large subunit joins amino acids according to specified instructions from the codon to form a protein (figure 5.23). This illustration shows just one triplet. There can be many triplets (hundreds or thousands) within a messenger, specifying many amino acid linkages.

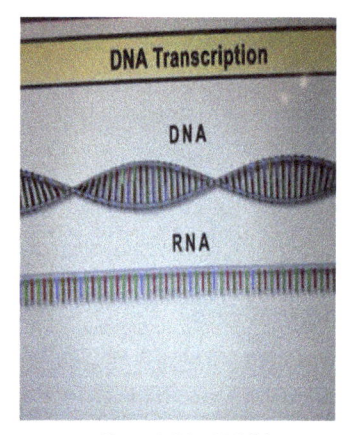

Fig. 5.22. DNA Transcription.

David Savada PhD, *Pritzker Family Foundation Professor of Biology, Claremont Colleges,* "Lecture *DNA Structure and Replication" Understanding Genetics,* The Great Courses. 2008 DVD

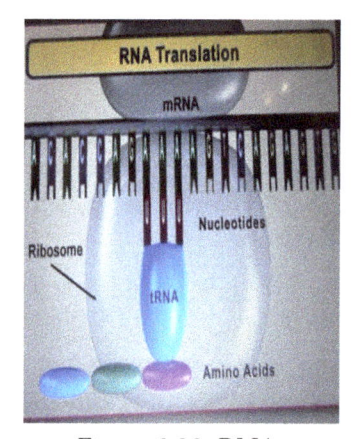

Figure 5.23. RNA Translation.

David Savada PhD, *Pritzker Family Foundation Professor of Biology, Claremont Colleges,* "Lecture *DNA Structure and Replication" Understanding Genetics,* The Great Courses. 2008 DVD

Proteins

So, what are proteins? Proteins are described in various ways—molecules, polymers, biomolecules, macromolecules, enzymes, or hormones. The bottom line is that proteins are chemical combinations used in the functions of humans. Since all species are composed of chemicals, the proteins are the products of the chemical factory in cells. A gene's DNA specifies the order and number of the amino acids that define a blueprint for the role the protein will play—one gene, one protein (figure 5.24).

Proteins are polymers (long chains of chemical *beads*) composed of monomers called amino acids. There are twenty different amino acids, varied by their chemicals. Each protein contains all twenty amino acids. Carbon and nitrogen are the two main chemicals in amino acids. Nitrogen links with hydrogen to make the amine group, and carbon links with oxygen to make the acids group. Humans lack the genetic capacity to make eight essential amino acids contained in the amine group. These eight essential amino acids must be eaten as part of a person's daily diet. Foods high in essential amino acids include meats, dairy products, seafood, eggs, grains, nuts, and some vegetables.

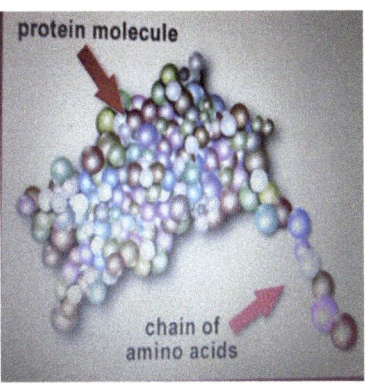

Fig. 5.24. Protein.

David Savada PhD, *Pritzker Family Foundation Professor of Biology, Claremont Colleges*, "Lecture *DNA Structure and Replication*" *Understanding Genetics,* The Great Courses. 2008 DVD

A long chain of amino acids varies from ten to one thousand monomers. A chain of two to fifty amino acids is called a peptide. Over fifty amino acids are considered a protein. Proteins are expressed as phenotypes.

There are two types of proteins: structural and enzyme. Structural proteins are the essential mechanism of human functions, good or bad. Enzymes perform as catalysts. Structural proteins fold into a three-dimensional shape as required for their role and as specified by DNA. Enzymes are proteins with specific catalyst functions and folded into complex shapes.

Summary

Indisputably, the brain is the most complex and magnificent organ in the human body. Its development through the first twenty weeks of gestation begins the creation of a unique human from the evolutionary genes and traits of past generations. Think of the mathematical combination of all the brain parts and processes. These define the complexity facing researchers and scientists.

The odd-looking structure of the neuron becomes an efficient design as the role of external and internal parts become understandable. Could it be that today's internet technology was copied from the brain's nervous system? The axons, dendrites, glial cells, cerebral spinal fluid, neuro-immune system, and blood-brain barrier are all vital to the external pathways and communication process.

Internal to the cell, DNA structure has been confirmed as genetic material in a double helix that contains two strands (one from the father and one from the mother) loosely connected by a hydrogen atom. These strands contain forty-four chromosomes in twenty-two autosome pairs. The chromosomes have an uneven distribution of 26,000 genes. It has been confirmed that the code language of DNA includes information and four chemical structures represented by the letters A, T, C, and G. These letters are always in pairs of A=T and C=G.

The use of this information requires a mechanism to convert the DNA chemical structure of A, T, C, and G into a protein chemical structure of amino acids. Deciphering the genetic code in 1961 led to understanding the processes of transcription, translation, and transportation to make proteins in the ribosome.

Proteins are the workforce whose makeup carries the communication within the brain and to the body. *Amino acids* are building blocks that form the individuality of a protein as well as influencing electrical signal capability.

The amazing progress made in the last fifty years is due to both the tremendous contribution from researchers and the benefits of advances in technology from achievements like the Apollo program, the microchip, computers, the genome and genetics, MRIs, PET scans with tracers, and now CRISPR/Cas9. The development of the microchip in the 1960s and its evolution to today's virtual machines and nanotechnology are providing the tools for tomorrow's therapies for treating AD. Chapter 6 will discuss how research evolved.

6

Alzheimer's Disease (AD) Research

Research involves many disciplines to achieve proof of concept. This chapter will discuss some of the disciplines and pathways along the way. The fundamental research model is in three segments. There is basic research, usually done by universities and academia. There is translational research that involves a relationship between government, academia, and industry, which aims to *translate* findings of basic research into medical practice and meaningful health outcomes. The final stage is industry (in the case of AD, it is pharmaceuticals) to demonstrate proof of concept through clinical trials.

In 1906, with the naming of AD, the only means available for research was the microscope and autopsies. Researchers used their knowledge of chemistry, biology, and physics to further their knowledge of AD.

Then in 1944, a new discipline became available as Oswald Avery performed experiments identifying DNA, and this gave birth to genetics. With advances in genetics, chromosomes, and genes were identified for AD. Cognitive diagnostic measuring tools evolved from psychiatric experience and became cognitive biomarkers for AD.

With the increase in lifespans and growing awareness of AD, advocates in 1974 influenced the creation of the National Institute of Aging, followed in 1980 by the Alzheimer's Association.

The beginning of the twenty-first century saw AD research benefit from the technology advances of the twentieth century as the delicate spinal tap became a normal clinical biomarker, along with magnetic resonance imaging (MRIs) and positron emission topography imaging (PET scans) with radioisotope ligands (tracers).

This chapter further explains the three disciplines along with the difficulties and uncertainties of the research scavenger hunt for cure, delay, and/or prevention of AD.

Research Model Threat

Historically, the research model has worked based on the medical and financial benefits outweighing the risks. A 2011 paradigm shift for AD could threaten the model as the paradigm shift's approach could face social and financial uncertainties due to length of time to determine AD interventions' efficacy, creation of public-private partnerships, patent ownership outcomes, and uncertainties for volunteers. [Ref. 20] Societal issues include drug affordability, insurance reimbursement, high cost of diagnostic, and biomarker test tools (CSF, PET scans and tracers, MRIs, DNA tests, and CRISPR/Cas9, etc.). How will public pre-symptomatic candidates (probably age forty-five to sixty-five) afford the cost for diagnostics and medical treatment if an intervention becomes FDA approved?

AD Basic Research—Academia

University laboratories have been guided by the amyloid cascade hypothesis to pursue beta and gamma secretase enzymes as AD therapeutic targets. In addition, they have evolved biomarkers to improve confidence in both the preclinical and clinical environment. Significant in these biomarkers are structural and functional MRIs and PET scans. Cerebrospinal fluid analysis provides another clinical biomarker through evaluations of amyloid beta peptides and the tau protein.

With completion of the Human Genome Project in 2003, this field is accelerating into a growth industry. From crops to oil spills to medicine, genetics is making significant contributions. The 2012 invention of CRISPR/Cas9 to modify DNA (to correct mutations that cause diseases) provides not only hope, but also societal concerns. *(See chapter 7 for more on CRISPR/Cas9.)*

Worldwide research laboratories are benefiting from ever improving technology such as computers for handling big data, nuclear medicine ligands (tracers) for PET scans, DNA sequencing systems for mutation detection and analysis, and improved transgenic animal models. These tools have supported the researcher's creativity to dig deeper and deeper into the complex problem of gaining more knowledge of the brain and its magnificent functionality. Each small piece of this unquantified problem can provide a career for any young researcher.

When studying the brain and AD, the amount of known knowledge is overwhelming. However, while studying, one gains the opinion that the surface of the total knowledge has just been scratched and that possibly only ten or twenty percent is known. It is as if we will never know everything.

Today's basic research is like a shotgun blast, going in all directions. A systematic integrated approach does not appear to be a near term option. This may be acceptable for the current state of knowledge. The creativity, dedication, and knowledge displayed in the thousands of yearly research reports are testimony to the collective talents of thousands of men and women in the research community. A caregiver like Bruce says, "Thank you and please continue your outstanding dedication and contribution."

AD Transitional Research

Transitional research is moving promising therapies from the laboratory to a clinical environment for proof of concept. This transition is not as easy as it may sound. Like the joy experienced at the birth of a newborn child, the excitement involved with a new

Alzheimer's therapy or biomarker often overlooks the development challenges (like a mother's nine-month pregnancy). Transitional research is exemplified by the development of today's PET scan technology. Prior to the introduction of a nuclear medicine tracer (Pittsburg Compound B-PiB) in 2004, the only certain identification of neuritic plaque and tangles was by autopsy after death. The PiB breakthrough now allows imaging of amyloid in a living human. Later followed by tau tracer AV 1451. (Ref. 47)

Researchers at the University of Pennsylvania introduced the concept that led to PET scans in the late 1950s. Their development of emission and transition instruments led to future topographic imaging equipment, developed in 1975 by researchers at Washington University in St. Louis. Meanwhile, researchers at Brookhaven National Laboratory were developing radiopharmaceuticals (radioactive tracers used for imaging). Brookhaven developed 2-fluoro-deoxy-D-glucose (2-FDG) that was demonstrated in 1976 at the University of Pennsylvania through a human volunteer. Years later, a University of Pittsburg research team, led by geriatric psychiatrist William E. Klunk and radiochemist Chester A. Mathis, developed many compound agents (radioactive isotopes) with suitable properties for use with PET scan imaging.

Through a partnership with the University in Uppsala, Sweden, Henry Engler conducted the first tests of these compound agents at the university in February 2002. PET scan images showed that the second compound tested attached to amyloid in areas of the cerebral cortex (previously known only through post-mortem examinations) to contain significant amyloid deposits. Henry Engler named the isotope Pittsburg Compound B (PiB). The initial human trial of PiB expanded to include sixteen AD subjects and nine cognitively normal controls. Results were published in 2004 in the Annals of Neurology. (Ref. 12)

PiB is a fluorescent element recorded by the PET scans imaging (figure 6.1). The half-life of this isotope permitted only twenty minutes for imaging. Therefore, the University of Pittsburg licensed GE healthcare to develop an agent (tracer) that would remain stable enough for clinical use. GE Healthcare's imaging agent, Flutemetamol, renamed Vizamyl, a F18-labeled ligand (tracer), received conditional approval from the Center of Medical Services (CMS) on September 27, 2013. (Ref. 19) The transitional research and development image in figure 6.1 shows a PiB PET scan of a patient with AD on the left and an elderly person with normal memory on the right. Areas of red and yellow show high concentrations of PiB in the brain and suggest high amounts of amyloid deposits in these areas. Because of this transitional research, patients with presymptomatic conditions are being identified. They are also pursuing solutions for measuring very small changes in both the disease and in evaluating patient cognitive changes.

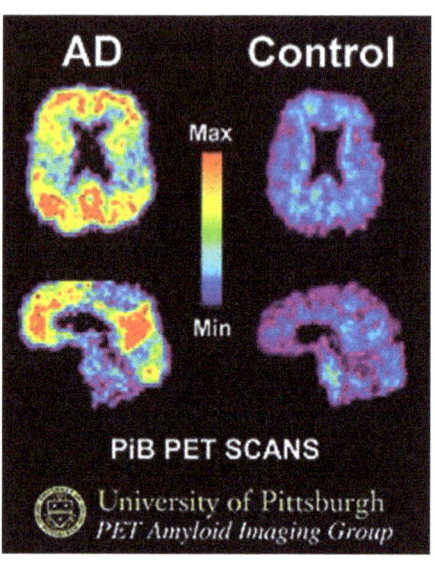

Fig. 6.1. PiB PET Scans.

Developmental Research

Pharmaceutical companies are still pursuing developmental research on various drug candidates, but they have redirected from volunteers with mild and moderate AD to volunteers with mild cognitive impairment (MCI) and, where possible, volunteers who can qualify with presymptomatic conditions. Pharmaceutical companies hope to find products that delay AD (as statins have for heart disease).

However, the real preclinical issue becomes benefits versus risks. Can a pharmaceutical company afford the investment risk of a ten- or twenty-year trial with current patent laws and potential government pressure to cut drug costs? Is this a threat to the paradigm shift and early prevention research for AD? A poignant question is "Why would anyone want to know they have AD a decade before they might develop symptoms if there is nothing they can do about it?" (Ref. 21)

A Lifetime of Alzheimer's Disease Research

Oswald Avery identified DNA in 1944, which advanced genetic research, led to the expansion of dementia and AD research of the 1970s and beyond. These genetic and dementia achievements add to the many twentieth century discoveries that made Bruce and Ethel thankful to be part of The *Lucky Few Generation: Between the Greatest Generation and the Baby Boom* (2008 book by Elwood Carlson).

Bruce's comment: So much AD knowledge gained and so many discoveries made with so little patient benefits. If there is one criticism for these years, it is promoting volunteer expectations relative to the overwhelming complexity of AD. Based on the following evidence, each reader can be his own judge. I believe the research community has done an excellent job in increasing its knowledge and understanding of the many AD issues. Unfortunately, there are just too many variables and issues associated with the one hundred billion neurons in the brain as well as social-political advocacy in an over-populated world. (Appendix C provides a list of key discoveries, findings, developments, and improvements that led to advancing both the medical knowledge and public awareness.)

The Oswald Avery 1944 experiment led to James Watson and Francis Crick's 1953 description of the double helix structure of DNA. Alfred Hershey and Martha Chase proved DNA was genetic material the same year, advancing the field of genetics. It provided the basis for translating genetic knowledge into the clinical research applications. This led to the tau protein extra cellular role in 1975, beta amyloid peptide in 1984, tau tangle in 1986, and the amyloid precursor protein (APP) gene in 1987.

Ethel's father (Dr. Howard Heinecke) had AD as did his father. Dr. Heinecke's 1992 death certificate identified cause of death as senile dementia (AD was not medically accepted then). His final year in nursing facilities was much different from today as they used physical restraint then. Major positive changes have occurred over the last thirty years, thanks to dedicated and probably unrecognizable researchers, along with advocacy organizations such as the Alzheimer's Association (1980) and others, including the Lou Ruvo "Keep Memory Alive" foundation (1995) in Las Vegas, Nevada.

As decade's roll by, knowledge builds on knowledge gained as with dementia and Alzheimer's. The identification of tau tangles, beta amyloid, and the APP gene found on chromosome 21, led to the belief that plaque and tangles found during brain autopsies were the cause of AD. Since the plaque preceded the tangles, there was a belief that inhibiting amyloid production and clearing the plaque might cure AD.

Fig. 6.2. The Amyloid Cascade Hypothesis. (Ref. 22 & 56)

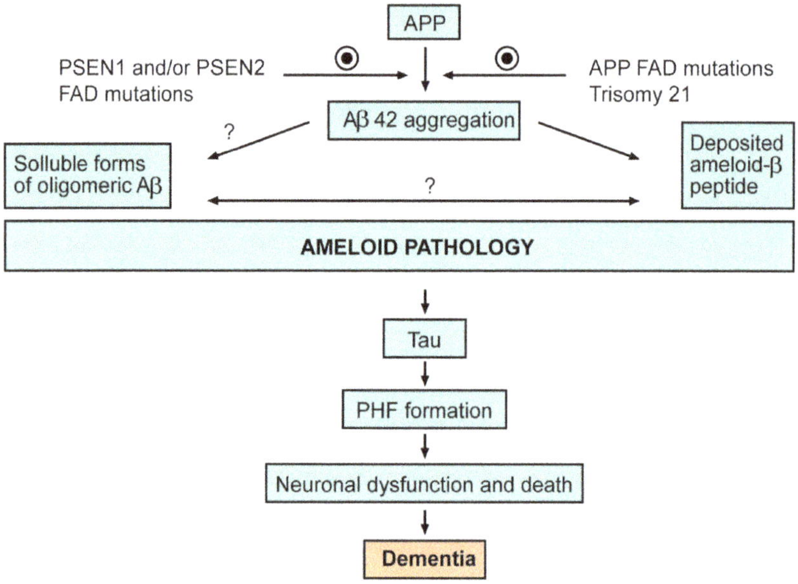

```
                           APP
PSEN1 and/or PSEN2    ⊙    ↓    ⊙    APP FAD mutations
FAD mutations              |         Trisomy 21
              ?     Aβ 42 aggregation
   ┌──────────────┐                  ┌──────────────┐
   │ Solluble forms│                 │  Deposited   │
   │of oligomeric Aβ│       ?         │  ameloid-β   │
   └──────────────┘                  │   peptide    │
                                     └──────────────┘
   ┌─────────────────────────────────────────────┐
   │            AMELOID PATHOLOGY                │
   └─────────────────────────────────────────────┘
                        ↓
                      ┌─────┐
                      │ Tau │
                      └─────┘
                        ↓
                ┌───────────────┐
                │ PHF formation │
                └───────────────┘
                        ↓
         ┌──────────────────────────────┐
         │ Neuronal dysfunction and death│
         └──────────────────────────────┘
                        ↓
                   ┌──────────┐
                   │ Dementia │
                   └──────────┘
```

The amyloid cascade hypothesis posits that the deposition of the amyloid-β peptide in the brain parenchyma (neurons and glia cells) is a crucial step that ultimately leads to AD. This hypothesis was first postulated twenty-five years ago and has been modified over the years as it has become clear that the correlation between dementia or other cognitive alterations as well as amyloid-β accumulation as plaque, is not linear.

Figure 6.2 is an illustration of the amyloid cascade hypothesis (ACH) as originally postulated in the 1980s. Bruce's explanation of figure 6.2 follows: *APP is the Amyloid Precursor Protein. PSEN1 and PSEN2 are two genes associated with Early Alzheimer's disease (patients around thirty-five years of age). APP FAD is familial Alzheimer's disease, where a mutation on the APP gene causes an excess production of amyloid. Trisomy 21 is Down syndrome.*

Down syndrome, first identified in 1862, has many of the progressive symptoms associated with AD. In 1959, the cause of Down syndrome was identified as a third chromosome 21. Chromosome 21 hosts the APP gene and results in the production of excessive amyloid in a Down patient's brain. Such excess is believed to be the contributor to AD progressive symptoms. (Ref. 46) Beta amyloid is a peptide with either forty or forty-two amino acids from APP. AB_{40} is the soluble form and found in the brain's extra cellular space. AB_{42} forms fibrils that become toxic and aggregate into plaque. AB_{40} is the greater amount and is cleared in cerebrospinal fluid (CSF) and through blood plasma.

An enzyme called gamma secretase cuts APP to form the beta amyloid peptide with forty-two amino acids (AB_{42}—center rectangle in figure 6.2). The left rectangle indicates oligomers in soluble form, where these oligomers diffuse from either AB_{40} or AB_{42}. An oligomer is a couple of dimers (two monomers) or a few monomers (monomer is an individual amino acid—figure 5.14) that separate from the beta amyloid peptide, become diffuse amyloid, and can aggregate to form plaque. Aging appears to either cause an over production of beta amyloid or a decrease in the process to clear beta amyloid from the brain in some people, thereby losing proper function to maintain a required amyloid balance. Either of these possibilities results in excess beta amyloid, which becomes toxic and through aggregation builds into plaque. Aggregative Stress (Figure 6.2) is a catchall for complicated biological action that is not totally understood. However, involved in the ACH process is that the oligomers can become toxic and proceed to create a plaque that is believed to be in the synaptic space (figure 5.10) or attaches to either an axon or dendrite. Paired helical fibrils (PHF) (fig. 6.2) indicate a breakdown of the tau protein which leads to neuronal dysfunction and death of the neuron.

Whether oligomer aggregation or plaque accumulation causes the tau protein to become dysfunctional is not known. Tau protein functions by facilitating the transfer of information from inside the nucleus through the membrane, either to an axon or from a dendrite. This can be like railroad tracks that allow a train to move between destinations.

ACH $_{(Ref. 56)}$ has been studied and pursued for a quarter of a century and is yet to be proven valid. Research complexity is vast. The focus has been on two enzymes, beta, and gamma secretase. Gamma secretase has had many failed drug candidates and still has major complexities. Beta secretase has taken longer to reach clinical trials (where they are now in 2017). However, due to unknown complexities, these may follow the path of gamma secretase—namely a scavenger hunt for finding the next clue.

Though clinical trials failed from 2002 to today (2017), the failures have only been part of the story. Since the optimism in 2001, a paradigm shift in 2011 recognized that the disease of volunteers with mild and moderate Alzheimer's were too advanced for candidate therapies to be successful, thereby refocusing strategy to delay symptoms before symptoms start. Despite many advances in knowledge, learning, and improved tools, uncertainties still existed in 2011 and even today. Along with the paradigm shift and the introduction of radioisotope tracers, new drug candidates are focusing on amyloid oligomers and monomers as well as developing tracers that could provide PET scan imaging as biomarkers. ACH, published in 1992, led to amyloid research domination over the next twenty-five years. Was this domination prudent or justifiable? You be the judge based on the following.

Tau Protein

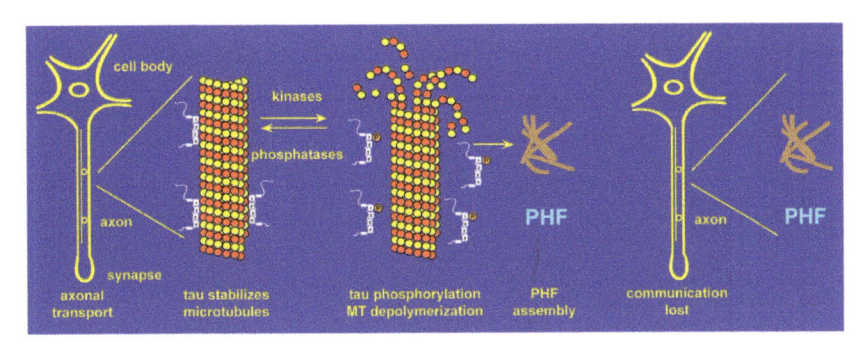

Fig. 6.3. Tau protein, microtubules & PHF

The tau protein linkage to neurofibrillary tangles was first made in 1986. The tau protein is produced (synthesized) from the Microtubule-Associated Protein Tau (MAPT) gene on chromosome 17. A main function of the tau protein is to modulate the stability of axonal microtubules (figure 6.3) within the axon where communication is processed through the axon to the synapse terminal. Hyperphosphorylation of tau causes abnormal inclusions that form paired helical fibers, which aggregate into insoluble tangles and disrupt communication. Eventually, affected neurons die, and the neurofibrillary tangles remain in extracellular space as tombstones of the cells destroyed by the disease. (Ref. 32) What causes phosphorylation to become hyperphosphorylation is unknown.

During early 2016, investigators, at the University of California, Berkeley, Helen Wills Neuroscience Institute, were able to use a novel PET tracer (AV-1451) to track the progression of tau protein pathology in volunteers with AD and normal controls. They found that higher quantities of tau in the medial temporal lobes of the brain were associated with greater decline in episodic memory. (Ref. 47) PET tracer images were also compatible with the view that tau inclusions first appear in the transentorhinal cortex, (Ref. 39) from where they spread to distant brain regions, given enough time. (Ref. 47) Tau-PET tracers have allowed researchers to confirm in vivo (living patients) Braak's postmortem neuropathology finding that tangle pathology spreads out of the medial temporal lobe into the neocortex as AD progresses (Ref. 47). This progression is due to an unknown mechanism of amyloid plaque. "Tau imaging is a transformational technology," commented Clifford Jack of the Mayo Clinic in Rochester, Minnesota. (Ref. 35)

"Aβ and tau are originally separated in space and time. The mechanisms that drive this synergy are not yet understood," said Gil Rabinovici at the University of California San Francisco Memory and Aging Center. Amyloid deposition starts in the neocortex and progresses over time to the medial temporal lobe. Plaques play a key role for the spread of tangles through the brain, only when amyloid has accumulated. (Ref. 35) Tau deposition in the medial temporal lobe increases with age regardless of the presence of Aβ, but the spread of tau to the neocortex is highly dependent on the copresence of amyloid pathology. (Ref. 35) When comparing Ethel's sixteen years of decline as described in chapter 3 to the Braak stages and symptoms, matches on a broad scale seem similar relative to behavior, progression, and time. Mapping tau pathology, with linkages to symptoms, behaviors, and stages, along with MMSE scores, might help in establishing the efficacy predictions of trial designs. It could also benefit caregiver's expectations *(more on au in chapters 7 and 8)*.

Evidence

Appendix C timeline suggests that dementia and Alzheimer's research began an acceleration about the mid-1980s. Was this acceleration a result of the attention and advocacy given by the National Institution on Aging (1974) and the Alzheimer's Association (1980)? The evidence (research reports) suggests the primary methodology during the last quarter of the twentieth century was autopsy analysis. A main thrust was to answer whether AD was a disease or just a continuation of the aging process. Increases in lifespan and AD awareness led researchers to developed methods to measure cognitive decline. Meanwhile a genetic mutation in the APP gene was identified as a hereditary cause of Familial Alzheimer's disease (FAD) in 1992. (Ref. 46)

In 1991, the husband and wife team Heiko Braak and Eva Braak (professors at the Institute of Clinical Neuroanatomy, Johann Wolfgang Goethe-University, Frankfurt am Main, Germany) published a *pivotal autopsy report* of their examinations of eighty-three demented and non-demented volunteered brains. (Ref. 39)

Results showed that tau inclusions form in a stereotypical fashion, allowing classification depending on where the inclusions are found and in what number. Their cross-sectional autopsy studies of tau pathology showed first deposits in transentorhinal cortex (stages I/II), followed by hippocampus (stages III/IV) and neocortex (stages V/VI)—Braak stages. They opined that loss of neurons in the transentorhinal cortex (EC) is the starting point for AD cognitive symptoms. (Ref. 39) *They concluded that AD begins many years before symptoms appear and that it is a very slow progressing disease.*

The entorhinal cortex (EC) (fig. 6.4) plays a crucial role as a gateway connecting the neocortex and the hippocampal formation. The EC is affected severely in AD. (Ref. 16)

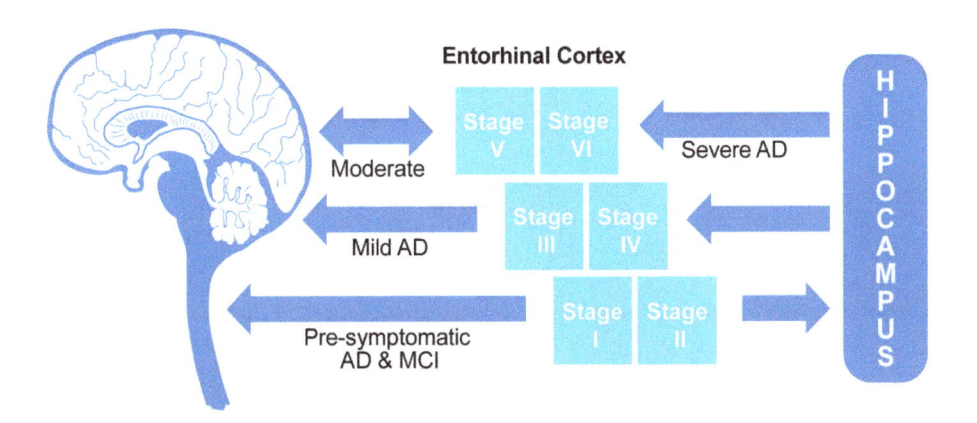

Fig. 6.4. Entorhinal Cortex.

Stage 2 of the EC (Braak stages) gives rise to the major source of the excitatory input to the hippocampus, and stage 4 receives major hippocampal input for transfer to the neocortex storage locations. In the cognitively normal individuals, ±650,000 neurons are in stage

2, one million neurons in stage 4, and seven million neurons in the entire EC. The number of neurons remained constant for cognitively normal people between sixty and ninety years of age. (Ref 16)

In a 1996 published report of autopsy tests of brains from twenty demented donors with various stages of AD, all of them had sufficient neurofibrillary tangles (NFTs) and senile plaques for the neuropathological diagnosis of AD. The group with the mildest clinically detectable dementia had 32 percent fewer EC neurons than the control group (a loss of over two million neurons). Decreases in individual's EC stages were even more dramatic, with the number of neurons in stage 2 decreasing by 60 percent and in stage 4 by 40 percent compared with controls. In the severe dementia cases, the number of neurons in stage 2 decreased by ±90 percent and the number of neurons in stage IV decreased by ±70 percent compared with controls. These results support the conclusion that a marked decrease of stage 2 neurons distinguishes even very mild AD from nondemented aging. (Ref. 16)

This 1996 report suggested interventions target presymptomatic conditions. Unfortunately, methods to determine such targets did not exist in 1996.

Bruce's comment: Lost neurons are not replaceable. Can reserve neurons become useful? Were trials with criteria of mild and moderate stage candidates automatically doomed?

In 1995, research laboratories received their first transgenic mice. This allowed labs to perform testing to build confidence for the safety and efficacy of an intervention. An immunotherapy synthetic beta amyloid vaccine in mice was reported a success in 1999. (Ref. 1) This led to a 2001 small clinical trial of eighty volunteers that proved successful for safety, along with a reported response by a volunteer's neuro-immune system. A rush to proceed with a phase 2 trial ended in a severe adverse event (SAE), which terminated the trial *(see chapter 4 and Appendix D—AN-1792)*. This vaccine demonstrated dissolution of amyloid plaque but had no effect on either tau or the neuro-degeneration process to end of life. However, two volunteers, who were at the very early mild stage and had their immune system activated, showed improved MMSE scores after one year. (Ref. 8)

Bruce found no follow-up reports on the two improved mild stage patients. Was this an opportunity lost? Was the stated improvement erroneous data? Could monitoring of the two volunteers from 2003 have provided a wealth of information whether plaque dissolution in an early stage may have delayed neurodegeneration and/or symptoms?

2011 Paradigm Shift (Ref. 20)—Research Redirection

With a decade of failed trials and a congressional push by former speaker of the House of Representative Newt Gingrich and former Supreme Court Justice Sandra Day O'Connor, national strategy changed to pursue a delay in AD rather than a cure.

AD is the only leading cause of death for which no disease-modifying therapy is currently available. Effective therapy for AD is a major unmet medical need. (Ref. 20) Recent disappointing trial results at the dementia stage of AD have raised multiple questions about the approaches to the development of disease-modifying agents. Converging evidence suggests that the *pathophysiological process* of AD begins ten to twenty years before the onset of AD symptoms.

The paradigm shift divided AD into two parts (AD-C and AD-P). AD-C is confirmation of AD by quantitative and qualitative biomarker data (symptomatic AD), and AD-P is the prodromal and MCI phase of AD (presymptomatic). Prodromal AD is either asymptomatic patients (risk factors such as ApoE4 without amyloid evidence) or patients with amyloid evidence from PET scans.

The concept that very early prodromal AD and mild cognitive impairment phases can be detected years before dementia becomes apparent has led to new guidelines that puts the clinical evolution of AD on a continuum that starts with a preclinical phase where the $A\beta$ *pathology of AD can be detected*, followed by *evidence of neurodegeneration*, both without any clinical findings, and evolve into the earliest clinical signs (Dubois et al., 2010).

Four general categories of anti-$A\beta$ therapy have been developed 1) agents that *decrease or modulate* $A\beta$ production to prevent or slow $A\beta$ aggregation and accumulation, 2) therapies that degrade or *enhance clearance* of Aβ aggregates, 3) aggregates therapies designed to *block* Aβ aggregates, and 4) therapies designed to *neutralize* toxic Aβ. (Ref. 20) Aβ aggregate accumulation begins in the brain because of reduced clearance/degradation or increased production. (Ref. 20)

Translational models suggest that anti-Aβ therapies may be highly effective if tested as agents to prevent or delay development of the disease or as therapies for asymptomatic patients with very early signs of AD pathology. (Ref. 20)

So why do we keep testing drugs aimed at the initial stages of the disease process in volunteers near the end-stage of the illness? (Ref. 25)

The National Institute on Aging and the Alzheimer's Association convened workgroups to provide recommendations for defining diagnostic criteria for preclinical AD. (Ref. 21) Recommendations in a May 2011 report (Ref. 21) provided a powerful description of the state of research, along with numerous uncertainties requiring resolution.

What is preclinical AD? The preclinical phase is now the major focus for research and funding. The workgroups (Ref. 21) defined a hypothetical dynamic biomarker needed for the preclinical phase. Currently nonexistent, such a biomarker was described to have the following features: (1) Aβ accumulation become abnormal first and a substantial Aβ load accumulates before the appearance of clinical symptoms. (*Bruce's comment: Possibly imaging technology can satisfy this.*) The lag phase between Aβ accumulation and clinical symptoms remains to be quantified, but current theories suggest that the lag may be for more than a decade. (*Bruce's comment: Makes the NAPA goal of prevention or delay by 2025 improbable.*) (2) Biomarkers of synaptic dysfunction, including PET scans and functional MRI (fMRI), may demonstrate abnormalities very early, particularly in *APOE* gene ε4 allele carriers. (*Bruce's comment: may or may not.*) (3) Structural MRI is thought to become abnormal a bit later as a marker of neuronal loss. (*Bruce's comment: a preclinical uncertainty.*) (4) No biomarker is static; rates of change, in each biomarker, change over time and follow a nonlinear time course, which is hypothesized to be sigmoid shaped. (*Bruce's comment: Concept to be proven.*) (5) Anatomic information from imaging biomarkers provides useful disease staging information in that the topography of disease-related imaging abnormalities changes in a characteristic manner with disease progression. (*Bruce's comment: Does this suggests a placebo signature profile could be modelled and let all patients participate in receiving the therapeutic agent.*)

Some of the needs and uncertainties identified in reports on the paradigm shift follow:

1. To move toward primary prevention, advances are needed in the ability to predict who is at very high risk for AD and in what time frame they might develop observable pathology and, subsequently, clinical symptoms.
2. Identification of additional factors that predict more precisely the risk for development of AD are needed. These are generically referred to as premorbid biomarkers and could be very useful in identifying an at-risk population for a primary prevention study.
3. In many scenarios, a fifteen- to twenty-year timeline would be the minimum time to test, possibly retest, and widely deploy an effective true primary prevention therapy or a therapy for the clearly asymptomatic preclinical stages of AD.
4. Without a biomarker and imaging-based stratification, mixed disease status at enrollment will complicate trial design by creating uncertainty regarding group size, length of trial, and potentially confounding results.
5. Is the duration of a primary or secondary prevention trial far longer than what the commercial sector is generally willing to entertain?
6. Does our current drug development environment need to revisit the legal policies that could discourage investment in primary prevention studies.
7. Are policies needed to transparently balance public health needs with private sector marketplace driven incentives?

So, how do you find volunteers with no symptoms until twenty years later and convince them to participate in trials with unproven human therapeutic results? In addition, where is the incentive to fund such risks, especially with biomarkers still evolving? This was the challenge undertaken by researchers during 2012 and 2013, resulting in the A4 clinical trial of December 2013.

Did the 2006 Australian Imaging, Biomarkers, and Lifestyle (AIBL) longitudinal cohort study with 1,822 participants—1,201 of them cognitively normal at the time begin the paradigm shift? These cohorts will become trial-ready for prevention trials (Ref. 34).

The following statement gives minimum realistic expectations: *Definitive studies are needed to (1) determine whether many asymptomatic individuals with evidence of AD-P are indeed destined to develop AD dementia, (2) elucidate the biomarkers and/or cognitive endo-phenotype that are most predictive of cognitive decline, and (3) determine whether intervention with potential disease-modifying therapies in the preclinical stages of AD will prevent dementia. These are likely to take more than a decade to accomplish fully.*

Bruce found the reports in References 20 and 21 to be powerfully realistic with a focus squarely on biology's basic research to explore the pathophysiology of amyloid accumulation to amyloid deposition and neuronal injury, along with confirmation of recommended biomarkers for AD-P.

The December 2013 clinical trial (referred to as A4) is the first trial based on the paradigm shift strategy of 2011. (Ref. 26) This trial introduces new tools that appear innovative but with potential issues and uncertainties. It seems to have incorporated the benefits of lessons learned and used the best available biomarker tools for measuring efficacy. Will this be enough?

The paradigm shift and switching focus to AD-P created issues involving patients and caregivers for which recognition is not currently obvious. This may contribute to the improbability of NAPA goal for delay and/or prevention by 2015. These include governance-associated issues with insurance coverage, reimbursement of test expenses, answers to questions like "Why should people volunteer?" (In fact, Bruce attempted to determine his ApoE alleles. His primary doctor prescribed an order to identify ApoE alleles. Medicare would not cover the blood test and analysis. Bruce's expense was $900.)

The Center for Medical Services (CMS) has denied coverage of FDG PET scan tracer agents. (Ref. 19) Such denial and a lack of CMS coverage of tests to identified gene alleles and mutations associated with AD are constraints by the government whereby the general population cannot afford to search their DNA, even though approved by the FDA to do so. Such issues become part of the decision process by preclinical candidates. Hopefully, CMS will reconsider their decisions, so all individuals are empowered and encouraged to determine their AD risks along with supporting the NAPA goal to treat or prevent AD by 2025.

Most encouraging is the scientific community's leadership. They are formulating the approach for the new concepts that include utilization of technology, biology, mathematical algorithms as well as correcting previous misjudgments. The efforts of these leaders have integrated the international community, which has stimulated international government support. So, what changed and what is better? The answers below will explore Lessons Learned and the present clinical and cognitive biomarkers.

Lessons Learned

The start of the twenty-first century began with unfortunate results of clinical trials but with a significant increase of knowledge. This knowledge, along with advances in technology such as magnetic resonance imaging (MRI), genetics, and positron emission topography (PET) radioisotope ligands (tracers) guided the 2011 paradigm shift.

Questions such as "Why do we keep testing drugs aimed at the initial stages of the disease process in patients at the end-stage of the illness?" [Ref. 22] led to a new clinical trial criterion that selects presymptomatic and mild cognitive impaired (MCI) candidates. Unfortunately, this new strategy took twenty years and many millions or billions of dollars to confirm earlier evidence [Refs. 16 & 39] as well as evidence indicated above.

Before MRIs and Pet scans, there was a report by Teresa Gómez-Isla et al, July 15, 1996, entitled, "Profound Loss of Layer II Entorhinal Cortex Neurons Occurs in Very Mild Alzheimer's disease." [Ref. 16]. As indicated above, this report indicated that nearly 50 percent of critical neurons in the medial temporal lobe memory circuits are already lost by the very mild stage of AD. Four major conclusions of the study were the following: (1) Normal cognitive patients (age sixty to ninety) showed no neuron loss. (2) By contrast, patients with very mild AD, who were at the threshold of clinical detection of AD at that time, showed severe loss. (This neuronal loss was so marked that it must have started well before onset of clinical symptoms.) (3) The neuron loss paralleled the known neurofibrillary tangles (NFT) formation. (4) The degree of neuronal loss paralleled the incidence of NFTs and neuritic plaques but not to diffuse plaques (beta amyloid, AB_{42}) without neuritic changes.

The study results highlighted the need to develop new diagnostic tests to predict the presymptomatic and very mild stages of AD before massive neuronal loss occurred and when therapeutic intervention might be most effective (Ref. 16)

Unfortunately, 1996 knowledge and technology were insufficient for presymptomatic trials. The Human Genome Project had not been completed and today's tools (MRIs and PET scans, etc.) were not available. Technology was limited. Knowledge was advancing and assets like the atomic microscope, big data, and autopsy brain banks were in the future. Population awareness and public pressure increased in 1994 with President Reagan's announcement that he was facing AD.

Since 2002, the string of disappointing clinical trial results has raised concerns about the current strategy for development of AD-modifying therapies. Three hypotheses explain these AD trial failures: (1) They targeted the wrong pathophysiological mechanisms, (2) drugs did not engage the intended targets in patients, and (3) drugs were hitting the right targets but doing so at the wrong stage of the disease. (Ref. 25) There should have been a fourth hypothesis: *Reliable cognitive biomarkers were unavailable to measure the required small incremental decline change.* Until a reliable surrogate biomarker is validated, the field must rely on clinical outcome measures that reflect cognitive function. (Ref. 28)

So, where is research today? Bapineuzumab, Crenezumab, Solanezumab, Gantenerumab, and Aducanumab clinical trials have all indicated small, undefined benefits in early stage volunteers despite questionable and unconfirmed results. Could these be positive indicators for the paradigm shift's delay and prevention? If these interventions prove to provide delay, the AD statin may be found.

A May 10, 2017 Reuters article, "Billions saved because FDA didn't rush approval of Alzheimer's drug" by Gene Emery, is an inappropriate, myopic, or political view of a questionable FDA decision. The article focused on cost and efficacy failure due to evaluating the wrong stage of the disease as opposed to assessing the positive subset results indicating a small benefit for a mild cohort group—the mild cognitive impairment (MCI) volunteers. Should Solanezumab have received a limited approval for patients with MCI and presymptomatic conditions as verified by PET scan tracers? With Solanezumab safety demonstrated, this would have been a proactive method of advancing the confidence of caregivers and patients that there is hope for delay and prevention.

However, such a decision would not only have involved the cost of Solanezumab but also the cost of PET scan tracers to be reimbursed by Medicare, Medicaid, and the insurance industry. Such reimbursements were denied in 2013 by the Center of Medical Services (CMS). (Ref. 19)

Did this Reuters article spin the data? Did the FDA save one hundred billion dollars, or increase billions, by allowing those with MCI, presymptomatic and/or risk factor conditions to progress past the point of no help (mild and moderate stages) as demonstrated by targeting the wrong stage of the disease? How many millions of patients will continue to decline based on this 2012 FDA decision not to approve Solanezumab until proof that they desire is provided? Hopefully by the A4 clinical trial with Solanezumab, currently targeted to end in 2020 (extended to 2022). Did the Affordable Care Act influence the FDA and CMS decisions because of medical reimbursements from the government and insurance as opposed to science and concerns for patients and caregivers? Did Reuters and the FDA assess the risk/reward consequence of the Solanezumab denial based on evidence provided by researchers during the 1990s that too many neurons were lost in the entorhinal cortex by very early mild AD, whereby intervention at such a stage is unlikely to be beneficial? (Refs. 16, 39) *If Solanezumab is successful in the A4 trial, how many millions of patients (worldwide) will have passed the point of intervention help during these lost years (2012–2023)? Was the FDA decision based on science risks and patient care or politics?*

Biomarkers

What are biomarkers? What are measuring tools? What is their contributive value? Blood tests provide biomarkers for the organs of the body. Hearing tests provide a biomarker for ears. Eye tests provide a biomarker for eyes. Blood pressure, thermometers, X-rays, ultrasounds, electro-cardiogram (EGK) all provide markers for the medical profession to assess a patient's condition. All these are noninvasive. They all have increments and ranges that define normal, when that norm breeches, and corrective action is needed. When norms breech, symptoms usually occur. Markers are determined from scientific evidence, received from the body's chemistry, along with access to the organs involved.

Scientific evidence is evolving for the brain as technology provides state of the art research tools to analyze data obtained both invasive cerebrospinal fluid (CSF) and PET scan tracers, along with noninvasive MRIs. Within constraints, these measuring tools are classified as biomarkers and are used in clinical trials. The data from these biomarkers provide evidence of the brain's neurodegenerative pathways and decline progression. Table 6.1 provides an indication of the purpose of the biomarkers in clinical trials.

Table 6.1. Clinical Biomarkers.

Tool	Biomarker	Purpose
Cerebral Spinal Fluid	Soluble Beta Amyloid AB40)	Oligomers, Dimers, Monomers
	Beta Amyloid Plaque (AB42)	Toxic Aggregations
	Tau Protein	Disease Decline
	Phospho Tau	Tauopathy
Magnetic Resonance Imaging	Structural Mapping	Location & Density
	Functional	Pathways & Area
	Volume	Atrophy Decline
PET Scan Imaging Tracers	Amyloid Tracers	Determine Amyloid
	TAU Protein Tracers	Tau Pathology
	Glia Cell Tracers (future??)	Immune System

In addition, cognitive measurements, of which there are many, have evolved from the neuropsychiatric profession. They are uniquely designed inquiries that request a subjective patient/caregiver response. Test design targets are functional areas of the brain, symptoms, behaviors, senses, and daily lifestyles that define a cognitive state from which to measure disease change, stages, and efficacy of interventions. These have proven reasonably successful from a broad subjective view.

Cognitive biomarkers collect data through specially designed verbal tests of episodic memory, executive functions, and behavioral symptoms. Biomarkers used in clinical trials must have FDA approval.

Biomarker research desperately needs a cost-effective breakthrough. The current clinical biomarkers are costly, intrusive, and limited for public use. Current cognitive biomarkers are unproven to detect small incremental changes that will be required for early presymptomatic detection and change.

With the advances in MRIs and PET scan technology, AD stages were redefined in 2011 to accommodate a hypothesis that the disease begins ten to twenty years before symptoms appear. Evidence showed that soluble amyloid remnants and plaque precede and are needed for the progression of tau tangles that produce neuronal injury and correlate to patient symptoms.

Therefore, using the new MRIs and PET scan tools to detect amyloid in the brain before symptoms appeared, AD was redefined to include a presymptomatic stage. This cohort group was now known as prodromal Alzheimer's disease. (Ref. 21) A registry of candidates for this group is an ongoing process. These candidates include those with hereditary or genetic issues or concerned volunteers. Using MRIs and PET scan tools, the registry is classified in three stages: (1) cohorts with no amyloid evidence, (2) cohorts with amyloid (prodromal), (3) cohorts with amyloid and onset of symptoms (MCI).

Clinical Biomarkers

Cerebrospinal fluid (CSF) measures beta amyloid and the tau protein. It is known that the AB_{40} peptide is found as soluble amyloid and the AB_{42} peptide as plaque. These peptides are analyzed from CSF as biomarkers. The lag phase between Aβ accumulation and clinical symptoms remains to be quantified, but current theories suggest that the lag may be for more than a decade.

Tau protein research has gained significant knowledge through the mapping of tau pathways (tauopathy) using PET scans with advanced ligands (nuclear tracers). (Refs. 31, 37) This research has formulated a belief that tau tangles cause the first cognitive symptoms of AD. However, what triggers the tau tangles is unknown, but increases in tau protein that are found in CSF become another indicator of disease progression and is a biomarker.

Magnetic resonance imaging (MRI) has made significant advances during the twenty-first century and is now a useful biomarker. What started as a general structural view of the brain, MRIs are now functional (fMRIs). When the patient verbalizes, the fMRI records the involved brain functions. Analysis of this data can determine an effect of amyloid plaque. MRIs are now focusing in on specific brain sections to measure changes over time.

Positron emission tomography (PET) scans have become a twenty-first century Alzheimer's tool that is proving extremely valuable. Since acceptance of PiB, after research publication in 2004, it has become a worldwide AD biomarker tool. Advances made in the nuclear medicines now identify changes in progression and specificity. The current A4 clinical trial is using florbetaben, trade name NeuraCeq, which is a diagnostic radioisotope agent (tracer), developed for routine clinical application to visualize beta amyloid in the brain.

Dominantly Inherited Alzheimer Network (DIAN), an international research partnership, started a very beneficial clinical trial in 2009. As implied, DIAN is a trial for volunteers whose past generations had a gene mutation that is strongly linked to AD through increased amyloid production. This international trial started in March 2009 and is ongoing. Through MRIs, PET scans, and biological fluids (CSF), the trial identifies and collects data that classifies volunteers as symptomatic, presymptomatic (mutation carriers), or noncarriers. DIAN has created data and tissue centers. Upon completion of developing secure access methodologies, these centers will provide researchers a vast source of data.

The difficulty in the field of AD is that we have not yet established a firm link between the appearance of any specific biomarker in asymptomatic individuals and the subsequent emergence of clinical symptomatology. (Ref. 21)

Cognitive Biomarkers

Clinical trials began in the twenty-first century with four principal cognitive test tools: Mini-Mental State Examination (MMSE), Alzheimer's Disease Assessment Scale-Cognitive Subscale (ADAS-Cog), Disability Assessment for Dementia (DAD), and

Neuropsychiatric Inventory (NPI). These tests are described below followed by Table 6.2, Assessment of Test Measurement Tools.

MMSE measures general cognitive functioning: orientation, memory, attention, concentration, naming, repetition, comprehension, and ability to create a sentence and to copy two intersecting polygons. Total score is from subscores. Totals range from zero to 30. Higher scores indicate better cognitive states. Neurologists use MMSE to monitor patient decline. Caregivers should obtain this test result at each visit as shown in chapter 3. Caregivers can anticipate behavioral changes relative to MMSE scores (not perfect but very helpful).

ADAS-Cog is a multi-item, objective measure of cognitive function. The scale evaluates memory, language, and praxis (the process by which a theory, lesson, or skill is enacted, embodied, or realized), with items such as orientation, word recall, word recognition, object identification, comprehension, and the completion of simple tasks. The ADAS-Cog consists of eleven parts as follows:

(1) *Word recall task:* A person is given three chances to recall as many words as possible from a list of ten words (short-memory test).

(2) *Name objects and fingers:* Several real objects are shown to the individual such as a flower, pencil and a comb, and the individual is asked to name them. The person then must state the name of each of the fingers on the hand such as pinky, thumb, etc.

(3) *Follow commands:* A person is asked to follow a series of simple but sometimes multi-step directions such as "Make a fist" and "Place the pencil on top of the card."

(4) *Constructional praxis:* This task involves showing the person four different shapes, progressively more difficult such as overlapping rectangles, and asking them to draw each one.

(5) *Ideational praxis:* The person is asked to pretend he has written a letter to himself, fold it, place it in the envelop,

seal the envelop, address it, and demonstrate where to place the stamp.
(6) *Orientation:* The person's orientation is measured by asking him what his first and last name are, the day of the week, date, month, year, season, time of day, and location.
(7) *Word recognition:* The participant is asked to read and try to remember a list of twelve words. Then, the participant is presented with those words along with several other words and asked if each word is one seen earlier or not.
(8) *Remembering test instructions:* The individual's ability to remember directions without reminders or with a limited number of reminders is assessed.
(9) *Spoken language ability:* Throughout the test, the participant's language ability to be understood is evaluated.
(10) *Word finding difficulty in spontaneous speech:* Throughout the test, the participant is assessed on word-finding ability during spontaneous conversation
(11) *Comprehension:* The person's ability to understand words and language over the course of the test is assessed.

The ADAS-Cog/11 ranged from 0 to 70 points, with higher scores indicating greater degree of impairment. A negative change from baseline indicates a decrease in cognitive impairment.

Bruce's comment: The ADAS-Cog has many subjective areas requiring not only the memory of the patient, but also the variations associated with different administrators. Broad use is OK, but use in clinical trials is questionable to demonstrate efficacy.

DAD measures instrumental and basic activities of daily living in patients with Alzheimer's disease (AD). The DAD is administered to volunteers' caregiver in the form of an interview. This scale assesses a volunteers' ability to initiate, plan, and perform activities related to hygiene, dressing, continence, eating, meal preparation, telephoning, going on an outing, finance, correspondence, medications, leisure, and housework. Each item can be scored as 1 = yes, 0 = no, not applicable = NA. A total score is obtained by adding the rating for each question and converting this total score out of 100. Higher scores indicate better function; a positive change from baseline indicates an improvement

NPI:12-domain is a patient or caregiver's assessment of behavioral disturbances occurring in dementia: delusions, hallucinations, agitation/aggression, depression/dysphoria, anxiety, elation/euphoria, apathy/indifference, disinhibition, irritability/lability, motor disturbance, appetite/eating, nighttime behavior. Severity (1=mild to 3=severe), frequency (1=occasionally to 4=very frequently) scales recorded for each domain; frequency and severity for each domain score (range 0-12). Total score=sum of each domain score (range 0–144); higher score=greater behavioral disturbances; negative change score from baseline=improvement.

Bruce's comments: The MMSE and DAD tests are often given by neurologists during an appointment. It provides them a guide as to how a patient is declining. Caregivers should request these scores at each visit to appreciate the stage of the patient along with future expectations.

Table 6.2 below provides a comparative assessment of the cognitive biomarkers described above.

Table 6.2 – Assessment of Cognitive Test Measurement Tools

Measured	Test Name	Test Type	Used By	Bruce's View
Functional Test	Disability Assessment for Dementia (DAD)	Forty questions for a caregiver to answer based on past two weeks. For decline: DAD & MMSE are comparable. This is objective data.	Clinical trial & neurologist	Caregiver's reply is subjective and flawed by two-week time. DAD is not finite enough for mild & moderate clinical trials of eighteen to thirty-six months.

Table 6.2 – Assessment of Cognitive Test Measurement Tools (CONT.)

Measured	Test Name	Test Type	Used By	Bruce's View
Cognitive Tests	Mini Mental State Exam (MMSE)	Set of questions for patient's decline. Range 30 to 0.	Neurologist, clinical trials & memory care	All these are good for long-term decline (ten to twenty years) but are ineffective for moderate patients & questionable for mild. A patient with MMSE score of 15 has lost too many neurons for improvement. Stage ranges are too broad. Subjective tests were possible cause of failed trials.
	Neuropsychological test battery (NTB) z-score	Patient is given nine psychological tests. Use questionable for MMSE below 10.	Neurologist & Clinical trials	
	AD Assessment Scale Cognitive Subscale (ADAS-Cog)	Language and memory are measured by eleven parts. Normal =5 MCI = 31	Clinical trials	

ADCS-PACC (Ref. 28)

Alzheimer Disease Cooperative Study–Presymptomatic Alzheimer Cognitive Composite (ADCS-PACC) test is the primary cognitive measure for the current A4 trial (first AD presymptomatic trial). Reference 28 was published in August 2014. (Ref. 28) ADCS-PACC combines tests that assess episodic memory, timed executive function, and global cognition. The tests were developed from cognitively normal volunteers from the ANDI and AIBL longitudinal trials along with ApoE4 group of volunteers.

Though results from the development trial data were very encouraging, the variable of subjective responses to survey questions introduce a level of uncertainty.

Cognitive Biomarker Issues

Though the cognitive biomarker tests used from 2000 through 2015 were the best available, the variables involved complicated the attainment of desirable clinical trial result, namely cure. In addition to the heterogeneity of mild and moderate volunteers, variables included differences in education, comingling known and unknown risk factors (ApoE4 and APP mutation), environment, lifestyle behaviors, and caregiver inputs. Assuming data handling and analysis a nonfactor, data results obviously varied from volunteers who had declined past the point of expecting to experience any improvement due to the loss of too many neurons. Could a more limited and specific target have found an intervention for delay at some point in decline? Three years of stability at a certain decline point (such as MMSE 20) might have been a measurable end-point and beneficial if successful.

In studies that have modeled the curve of cognitive change versus time, the preclinical trajectory suggests not only a long and slow rate of presymptomatic change, but also a period of acceleration of performance decrement that may begin several years before MCI onset. (Ref. 21)

The data obtained during this period (2000–2015) may have value, for linking test scores ranges, to cognitive decline symptoms, to benefit families and caregivers dealing with everyday management of a patient. Chapter 3 addresses this from Bruce's experience with Ethel using MMSE scores relative to Ethel's cognitive symptoms and behavior.

Despite the existence of multiple studies spanning thousands of participants, the promise of both subjective and objective cognitive measures for assessing risk of progression to AD in individual elders has not yet been fully realized. (Ref. 21) Cognitive assessments are very challenging and with uncertainties, especially when small incremental change is required to determine efficacy. Combining biomarkers with measures sensitive to detecting very subtle cognitive decline are clearly needed. (Ref. 21) Will it be acceptable to claim efficacy due to disease process delays and decline delays based on subjective behavior changes?

From a caregiver and patient view, a positive gain would be elimination of the placebo methodology and develop a signature profile of the disease decline process to measure against, thereby allowing 100 percent participation in clinical trials.

A Research Target Example

This example from basic research to an attempt to reach the market provides a view of the cooperation between academia and industry, along with risks that pharmaceutical companies take, and the eventual cost of drugs.

The drug selected for the example is currently continuing its pursuit to the market. For sixteen years, Eli Lilly has been funding this therapy. It started in the laboratory as m266 and then transitioned into a trial as LY2062430 and finally named Solanezumab. The "mab" identifies it as a monoclonal antibody. As indicated before, monoclonal antibodies detect and purify a target substance by attaching to it. In the case of Solanezumab, the target is soluble amyloid. Purification would be like removing excess amounts from the brain and either preventing or delaying aggregation to plaque and possibly tauopathy.

March 2001: Basic research was ongoing on Aβ antibody m266 in collaboration between Eli Lilly and Washington University in St. Louis. It was reported that "peripheral anti-Aβ antibody alters CNS and plasma Aβ clearance and decreases brain Aβ burden in a mouse model of AD" (Authors: Ronald B. DeMattos, Kelly R. Bales, David J. Cummins, Jean-Cosme Dodart, Steven M. Paul, and David M. Holtzman).

May 2006: Eli Lilly transitioned and renamed the m266 antibody to LY2062430 and initiated a clinical trial: Effects of LY2062430 in Subjects with Mild-to-Moderate Alzheimer's Disease and in Healthy Volunteers (NCT00329082). The purpose was to study its safety in twenty-five healthy volunteers.

October 2006: A phase 2 safety trial of LY2062430 began. Enrollment was sixty-five, and it was determined to be safe.

May 2009: LY2062430 was retitled to Solanezumab, and a phase 3 clinical trial began: Effect of LY2062430 on the Progression of Alzheimer's Disease (EXPEDITION) (NCT00905372). Enrollment was one thousand, and efficacy was not attained. *This could be an example of the right drug but targeting the wrong stage (mild and moderate) of the disease.*

July 2013: Progress of Mild Alzheimer's Disease in Participants on Solanezumab versus Placebo (EXPEDITION 3—NCT01900665) Enrollment was 2,100. This trial was for volunteers with mild stage AD and with a target completion of October 2020 (extended to 2022). Eli Lilly terminated the trial in November 2016.

December 2013: Clinical Trial of Solanezumab for Older Individuals Who May be at Risk for Memory Loss (A4)—(NCT02008357) began. Enrollment was 1,150. This is a current trial, designed and predicated on lessons learned from failed trials. Target completion is April 2020. In June 2017, A4 researchers decided to quadruple the dose of Solanezumab from 400 to 1,600 mg, given intravenously every four weeks. In addition to the dosage change, the A4 study will lengthen by seventy-two weeks for a total duration of more than four and a half years. (Ref. 48) This extends the trial completion to March 2022, and with an analysis and approval cycle, a market expectation might be 2023. Even with success for delay, it could take another undefined period to prove prevention.

May 2016: Clinical Trial NCT02760602 began for a Study of Solanezumab (LY2062430) in Participants with Prodromal Alzheimer's Disease (Expedition PRO*). (*Trial was terminated June 2017.)

Only the A4 trial is current with a target completion of 2022. The basic research for the therapy in this trial began in 2001. This trial is pushing the state-of-the-art. The volunteers are people with an indication of AD, but without obvious symptoms. The lack of efficacy in the May 2009 trial appeared to be due to volunteers with a moderate stage of the disease, which had advanced too far for any benefit. In 2016, Lilly announced it would not pursue FDA approval of Solanezumab for mild AD. (Ref. 45) Therefore, Eli Lilly targeted pre-symptomatic volunteers in the December 2013 trial (A4) and volunteers without symptoms, who may or may not develop AD in the May 2016 trial (DIAN).

Was Eli Lilly's goal to prevent or delay the disease and reach the market with a therapeutic product like the use of statins in cardiovascular disease? If Solanezumab provides delay and becomes approved by the FDA, Eli Lilly will have invested over twenty years of research for a seventeen-year patent. *Bruce believes Eli Lilly's intentions are more than profits. Will anyone remember this effort if not successful?*

Summary

Over the last twenty-five years, research has progressed from postmortem autopsy analysis to positron emission topography (PET) imaging using nuclear medicine's radioisotope agents to analyze amyloid and tau in living humans. The perspective of this achievement has been somewhat masked by the well-intended push to find a quick cure based on the 1992 amyloid cascade hypothesis. These intervening years added significant assets such as transgenic mice, a vaccine trial that cleared amyloid plaque without delaying neurodegeneration, monoclonal antibodies trials that may have hit the right targets but at the wrong stage of the disease and tools such as MRIs, brain banks, DIAN, ANDI, AIBL, the Human Genome Project, PET Tracers, Alzheimer's in a Dish, and CRISPR/Cas9.

A 2011 paradigm shift from seeking a cure to delay and prevention appears to have been the right direction while gaining more knowledge. The 2011 National Alzheimer's Project Act (NAPA) provided congressional recognition that a problem exists. Advances in technology and genetics continue to provide encouragement. The balance between biological scientific advances and realistic acceptance by social advocates could improve or impede chances of breakthroughs.

People concerned today about AD should not expect a cure during their lifetime. They should focus their efforts on delay through active lifestyle with a good diet program. This should start as early as possible. A daily routine of exercise and diet should be in place at the age of fifty. They should strive to maintain good health to avoid putting chemical drugs into their bodies and brains and allow the immune systems (both brain and body) to function with minimum interference from antibiotics or recreational drugs. Until researchers gain more knowledge, the natural immune systems offer the best defense, especially if maintained through excellent health. AD patients and caregivers should follow the A4 clinical trials and hope Solanezumab is successful for delaying AD.

The transfer of DNA instructions to create a protein was discovered as a messenger RNA in 1959, which transported a codon (a 1961 developed code method that takes a DNA instruction and identifies the amino acids needed by a protein). This led to the genetic code. The Human Genome Project (HGP) proposed in 1984, started in 1990, and was completed in 2003. The project's DNA sequencing was aided by technology from Illumina Corporation, a 1998 start-up company. Since completion of the HGP, genetic research has been searching for risk genes and mutations. This expanding field saw CRISPR/Cas9 introduced in 2012. [Ref. 33] This new tool demonstrated a laboratory correction of mutations in DNA sequences. *(Chapter 7 will cover Genetics—Great Promise for the Future).*

Even with fabulous breakthroughs in technology and genetics, a recent report of a possible blood test to determine AD could become the best discovery. Without such a breakthrough, general population diagnostic cost may be prohibitive. Reimbursement of cost for current PET scan tracers has been denied by the center for medical services (CMS) [Ref. 19] These tracers are the current diagnostic methods for Prodromal AD.

The biomarker measuring issue is that blood provides the cost-effective ability to use chemistry and biology to define and measure problems. The neurons in the brain also use chemicals and biological principles, along with genetics. Thus far, mechanisms have not been discovered to analyze the chemical, biological, and genetics norms for the brain's neurons. CSF, considered invasive, is providing evolving evidence, and may discover future reliable norms like blood. Can MRIs and PET scans differentiate one hundred billion neuron's nuclei that contain over billions of subparts? That leaves genetics as the best opportunity through evolving technology and science, along with DNA sequencing and big data analysis to provide a definitive biomarker. Chapter 7 identifies some hope for the future with mathematical modeling and big data research.

Cognitive assessment, though improving clinical markers, is very challenging and with uncertainties, especially when small incremental change is required to determine efficacy. Will it become FDA acceptable to claim efficacy based on progression and decline delays relative to subjective behavior changes?

From a caregiver and patient's viewpoint, a positive gain would be elimination of a clinical trial placebo design criteria and utilize mathematical modeling advances along with decades of clinical and longitudinal trial data to develop signature profiles of AD disease decline processes to measure against, thereby allowing 100 percent participation in clinical trials.

7

The Future

What does the future hold for Alzheimer's disease (AD)—*hope, promises, delay, prevention, or cure*? These are all wants. What is reality? This chapter addresses moving research targets that are being pursued with evolving knowledge and tools. This evolution will probably make much of this chapter obsolete in twenty years. Hopefully the time it takes from the laboratory to market (currently estimated at sixteen years) will be significantly reduced during those twenty years.

The United States strategic outlook changed in 2011 from pursuing a cure to finding interventions that can delay and/or prevent the disease. Will continual research advances provide the knowledge necessary to achieve delay, prevention, and/or cure? The bottom line is *"Que Sera, Sera—Whatever will be, will be."*

A caregiver's common-sense view, based on research reports and applying an engineering background to problem solving, is offered by Bruce with the utmost respect for the many researchers, pharmaceutical companies, and organizations which are exploring the unknown (like Lewis and Clark) and contributing to the overall AD effort. Their knowledge, as reported in PubMed, provides educational material, which is appreciated. As each group may have a focus and priority with their own interests, so do caregivers, families, and Bruce.

Bruce's Perceived Issues

AD is not only biologically and chemically complex, but governance is also equally complex with its role in social, economic, political, and leadership variables. Will governance advance or impede future research efforts? (Ref. 19, 53, 61, 62) Though the twentieth century saw an unbelievable increase in knowledge, there are still many unresolved issues available for research. After over twenty-five years of pursuing the amyloid cascade hypothesis (ACH) without confirmation, there are both doubters and supporters. (Refs. 20 & 23) Addressing presymptomatic conditions may resolve this issue.

Bruce's suggests the following issues still need to be pursued by research:

1. *Additional knowledge is needed to design and validate a truly disease-modifying treatment.* (Ref. 24)
2. *ApoE4 risk factor: Will CRISPR/Cas9 be allowed to change mutated genes and the E4 allele to an E2 or E3? Will governance, cost, and social-political concerns impede such progress?*
3. *Biomarkers:*
   a. *Until a reliable surrogate biomarker is validated, clinical efficacy must rely on outcome measures that reflect subjective cognitive data* . (Ref. 28)
   b. *Very small incremental change from a reference baseline is desperately needed and the key to determining efficacy.*
   c. *Correlating biomarker analysis to symptom decline is also a patient/caregiver need. How will this be done in AD-P?*
   d. *Finding a cost-effective diagnosis biomarker is of the essence.*
4. *Presymptomatic candidates: What are the uncertainties? Who is selected? What determines efficacy? Can accurate efficacy be predicted? How will efficacy be measured? What is a baseline? Will MRIs and PET scan technology advances solve these issues?*

5. *Brain's immune system: Does it contribute positively or negatively? Who knows?*
6. *Genetics: Can genetic benefits and solutions find public acceptance?*
7. *Mitochondria: What role does mitochondria's energy producing source for neurons play in aging and AD?*
8. *Patients-Caregivers: Can advanced mathematics, artificial intelligence computer modeling, and simulations provide signature profiles, from which to measure against and eliminate the current need for a placebo cohort group? Can the FDA accept such advances?*
9. *Will these issues be part of future research?*

Uncertain State of Research

Decades of failed clinical trials have left Alzheimer's research with many uncertainties and questions such as the following:

1. Since amyloid plaque does not cause AD, what elusive role does it play?
2. Will causes for $A\beta_{42}$ elevation in most individuals with late-onset AD be found? (Ref. 24)
3. What initiates amyloid plaque fifteen to twenty years before AD symptoms appear? Why do some people proceed to AD and others do not?
4. Will questions about pathogenic mechanisms remain unanswered? (Ref. 24)
5. How many uncertain mechanisms (pathogenic, gene mutations, lifestyle, aging, neuro-immune system anomalies, hereditary genes, or something else) will be resolved in the next ten years?
6. What causes hyperphosphorylation of tau protein?
7. What is the mechanism linking tau to the amyloid cascade hypothesis?

8. What role does the immune system have in AD in relation to brain, body and glia cells?
9. Could CSF tau measurements provide meaningful data for pathway progression, tangles, hyperphosphorylation, and a normal baseline?
10. Can CSF tau measurements be related to AD symptoms?
11. How long will it be before very small incremental changes can be non-subjectively, cost-effectively, and accurately measured?
12. Will modeling, artificial intelligence, virtual reality and advance technology provide guidance for AD interventions?

These uncertainties, and probably many others, provide the challenges not only for all phases of research but also for government leadership and stakeholders.

The above uncertainties are only some of the research challenges. Since Alois Alzheimer identified plaque, fibrils, and tangles over a hundred years ago, knowledge of AD has increased like a child growing and learning. Will continued advances in knowledge and new discoveries provide intervention to avoid the oncoming AD tsunami? In the following pages, Bruce discusses possibilities for amyloid, amyloid cascade hypothesis, tau, biomarkers, genetics, CRISPR/Cas9, lifestyle, normal aging, caregiving, governance, reality predictions, and thinking outside the box.

Amyloid

The amyloid precursor protein (APP) is the primary protein for late onset AD (est. sixty-five years and older). A mutation in the gene causes an excess of brain amyloid. (Ref. 46)

Who has this gene mutation? Was it inherited? If not, how does it mutate? Can it be changed in the future? Will change cause adverse events elsewhere? Mutation changes are currently in basic genetic research and seem to be candidates for future intervention research, not only for the APP in AD, but other mutations in all dementia as well as normal aging. What will be known by 2033? (Bruce will be one hundred then.)

Excess beta amyloid (AB_{42}) becomes toxic and aggregates into plaque in the brain's extracellular space. The plaque is believed to interrupt synapses and attach to dendrites and axons of the neuron. Will future research determine the impact plaque has on synapses, axons, and dendrites? Could plaque be the accelerator of tau and the missing link? If so, how does it happen? If not, who can find this missing link between beta amyloid and tau? What will we know by 2033?

The AB_{42} vaccine, used in the 2001 AN-1792 failed clinical trial (Appendix D), triggered the immune system in some volunteers, who had plaque disrupted from their neurons but not cleared from their brains. (AB42 dissolved into AB40 but was not cleared.) They had no cognitive benefit and continued to decline in a similar manner as placebo patients. Two separate researchers opined that the disease had advanced too far and that if addressed at the beginning symptomatic point or earlier, the immune system may have been able to prevent the plaque aggregation and theoretically delay the start of cognitive symptoms and decline. [Ref. 25] Is a vaccine a future possibility?

Prodromal AD trials are now being attempted (a decade and a half later), with a search for volunteers who have presymptomatic conditions to determine if the disease can be delayed. [Ref. 26] Currently there are several uncertainties with this pursuit, namely the need for a tool to measure cognitive changes, a new criterion for selecting candidates, a criterion for efficacy, and, finally, determining if beta amyloid is the right target.

As of 2011, four general intervention categories of anti-Aβ therapy have been proposed: (1) agents that inhibit or modulate Aβ production in a manner that is designed to prevent or slow Aβ aggregation and accumulation; (2) therapies that degrade or enhance clearance of Aβ aggregates to improve the immune system's removal effectiveness; (3) therapies designed to block Aβ aggregation, thus preventing plaque; and (4) therapies designed to neutralize toxic Aβ aggregates. [Ref. 20]

Will the future of amyloid be determined by five clinical trials between 2014 and 2022? These trials are now targeting people with *no indication of amyloid* (or those who have *amyloid but no symptoms*) and those who have *mild cognitive impairment (MCI)*. Three trials include promising drugs, in theory, to clear amyloid from the brain: Solanezumab (2014–2022), Crenezumab (2016–2021), and Aducanumab (2015–2022). All three drugs clear amyloid but based on different methods. Two trial drugs, Elenbecestat (2016–2020) and Lanabecestat (2016–2021) inhibit the beta secretase enzyme from initiating the beta amyloid peptide (AB) (see figure 2.2).

Will amyloid be proven to initiate the cascade to AD? Will a cost-effective, nonsubjective, precise, diagnostic biomarker be discovered to measure small incremental change? Will PET scan radioisotopes imaging agents be expanded to associate symptoms to decline change? Answer to these and other questions will be future pursuits.

Current basic research studies into the biological structure of amyloid plaque may provide future understanding of the many plaque formations, their functions, along with their pathology. Worldwide application of chemistry and physics advance technologies are providing the capability to dig deeper in amyloid. Could the link to tau be near?

The Amyloid Cascade Hypothesis

What is the future of this hypothesis? The hypothesis (figure 6.2) lacks confirmation despite over twenty-five years of clinical trials. The results of the 2001 AN-1792 trial provided strong evidence that amyloid plaque may be only a promoter, not the cause of AD. Later evidence correlated cognitive decline symptoms with tau tangles. Recent evidence indicates acceleration in tauopathy when amyloid is present. Is this the cascade effect? Without an amyloid to tau linkage mechanism, the hypothesis remains unconfirmed.

Should the hypothesis continue as a leading research-funding allocation? This is a debatable question. Recent advances in technology (PET scans) have provided evidence to support a presymptomatic strategy showing that amyloid can appear in the brain ten to twenty years before symptoms appear. This presymptomatic strategy proposes that amyloid is an upstream occurrence, and that neurofibrillary tangles (NFTs) that cause injury to neurons and initiate symptoms occur downstream via the tau protein. (Ref. 36)

Until more knowledge solves this mystery, the current strategy is to attempt limiting tau pathology by preventing amyloid from intensifying and accelerating. This new strategy continues to support the amyloid cascade hypothesis with the objective of finding an intervention to delay AD through prevention of amyloid aggregation into plaque during presymptomatic years.

A failed 2014 clinical trial of Eli Lilly drug candidate semagacestat (Ref. 30) created doubts about the amyloid cascade hypothesis that led Bart DeStrooper of KU Leuven (university), Belgium, to defend the hypothesis in a leading-edge essay in the November 6, 2014, issue of *Cell*. (Ref. 29)

Professor DeStrooper struck a nerve, and a probing discussion ensued on Alzforum. (Ref. 30) Many from academia, industry, and clinicians commented. The inputs offered varying opinions with many favorable views to continue the ongoing research (scavenger hunt) to gain a better understand of the gamma secretase enzyme. Significant from all the comments by top researchers is the amount that is not known about gamma secretase enzyme after decades of research by these major contributors to the amyloid cascade hypothesis. Even with continued academic research, the comments led one to believe it will take another decade to reach a point where industry may want to commit resources to renew their venture into clinical trials.

Tau

The tau protein provides a communication mechanism (figure 7.1) from inside a neuron's nucleus through neuron's external mechanisms (axons and dendrites). Tau normally provides structural support for the axon's microtubule (figure 7.1). As tau becomes hyperphosphorylated, the support breaks and forms paired helical pairs

(HP). These helical pairs become toxic and aggregate into structural neurofibrillary tangles (figure 6.3) that eventually cause the neuronal injury and death. An increase in this dysfunction process correlates with symptomatic cognitive decline.

Uncertainties numbers 6, 7, 9, and 10 below are obvious future tau research opportunities and could provide a full agenda for any researcher.

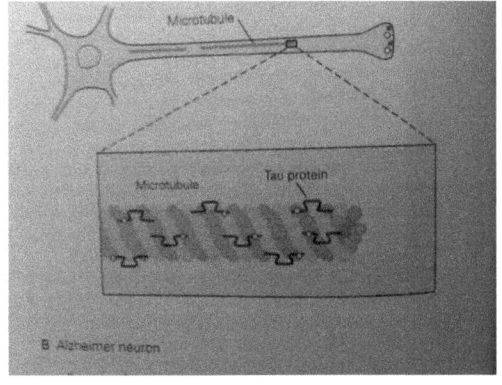

Fig 7.1. Normal Tau Microtubule in AD.

Uncertainty #6: What causes hyperphosphorylation of tau protein? Does lack of research material indicate the complexities in pursuing the answer to this question? Could amyloid plaque be involved? Can genetics help? How does NAPA Council view this relative to both AD and the tau mutation associated with frontotemporal dementia? This is just one of many uncertainties that need to be addressed with limited funding resources.

Uncertainty #7: What is the mechanism linking amyloid plaque to tau and the amyloid cascade hypothesis? Can PET scan imaging with AV-1451 tracer solve this mystery soon? Could an in-depth biology analysis of amyloid plaque's trigger of tau pathology be an expedited study?

Uncertainty #9: Could CSF tau measurements provide meaningful data for pathway progression, tangles, hyperphosphorylation, and a normal baseline? Comparing CSF tau measurements with PET scan imaging and MRIs could provide valuable analysis of CSF data and should be a future expectation.

Uncertainty #10: Can CSF tau measurements be related to AD symptoms? AD progresses at varying rates even among people who are at the same clinical stage. Because of this, trials need to enroll many participants to see a statistically significant slowing of progression. Could enrolling people based on their degree of tau pathology make cohorts more homogenous and trials more efficient? Modeling data demonstrated a rationale for using Braak stage as an entry point or a covariant for such trial participants. For future real-world trials, Braak stage could be determined by tau PET imaging. (Ref. 55) Could the A4 trial attempt to establish this by comparing resultant data of CSF measurement to amyloid and tau PET scan levels for each collection period? Could ANDI establish such data analysis with cognitive test data?

Is the current 2017 focus of pursuing therapeutic intervention of amyloid and tau the right strategy? The current strategy of presymptomatic intervention appears appropriate based on evidence that AD begins decades before symptoms appear. Once symptoms appear, neuron loss is too great to prevent disease progression. It appears that until the mystery of why and how beta amyloid accelerates the tau pathology and eventual neuron death that finding an intervention to delay such acceleration might need more time. If the scientific community can succeed in a decade to gain knowledge to resolve the current unknowns and uncertainties, some baby boomers and/or millennial generations may possibly realize delaying symptoms.

Tau tangles have been identified with dendrites. There is little or no reporting of this tauopathy. Should researchers select a certain function or action (such as turning on the TV) identify the genes and processes that are involved and study it as a closed-loop system to determine how it can be modeled on a computer? Could brain banks, longitudinal data, MRIs, and PET scan imaging provide source material? Yes, this is "outside the box," but such complex modeling could become future diagnostic medical tools.

Biomarkers

Biomarkers *lack a cost efficient, noninvasive method* to measure small incremental changes to diagnose AD and measure decline. There are two areas of concern until such a biomarker is discovered. Near term concern is research and clinical trials. Longer term concern is cost impact for public diagnostics, if a drug succeeds.

Many biomarkers, used now in clinical trials, provide data with a very high level of confidence. However, these are broad indicators, invasive, very costly, and mainly limited to clinical trials. Clinical trial biomarkers, mainly cerebral spinal fluid (CSF), MRIs, and PET scans, provide a wealth of data for research analysis and are continually improving. Possibly, one day, they may even succeed at measuring small changes, but cost is prohibitive for general population diagnostic use. Until a reliable surrogate biomarker is validated, the field must rely on clinical outcome measures that reflect cognitive function. [Ref. 28]

To move toward primary prevention, the *ability is needed to predict* who is at very high risk for AD and in what period this might develop observable and measurable pathology as well as subsequent clinical symptoms. Current evidence indicates increased risk for the progression of preclinical AD to MCI, and MCI to AD, but this evidence does not provide information regarding the onset of pathology. Even presence of an APOE-4 genotype only indicates increased risk or earlier age of onset but fails to provide precise information with respect to timing of disease onset. Identification of additional tools is needed that *predict more precisely* the risk for development of AD. Such tools may be referred to as *premorbid biomarkers* and could be very useful in identifying an at-risk population for a primary prevention study. [Ref. 20] Unfortunately, *such premorbid biomarkers are not currently available*. In 2011, the extent to which biomarkers of AD-P could predict a cognitively normal individual's subsequent clinical course remained for future clarification. (Ref. 21)

The 2011 paradigm shift to AD-P trials (Asymptomatic and Prodromal candidates) created concern for cohort selection and efficacy criteria. Presymptomatic data is either nonexistent or limited. Clinical biomarkers (tau and AB from CSF, MRIs, PET scans, and autopsies) were primarily based on symptomatic patients at various stages of AD.

Needing better cognitive biomarkers, a new cognitive test was developed during 2012 and 2013. This test, *Alzheimer's Disease Cooperative Study-Preclinical Alzheimer's Cognitive Composite (ADCS-PACC)*, utilized statistical techniques of prior data. ADCS-PACC is a composite of well-validated neuropsychological tests that were selected specifically because of their sensitivity in tracking the earliest evidence of decline, from normal to subtly abnormal cognitive performance. ADCS-PACC includes four tests: a picture-word list learning test, a paragraph recall test, a timed executive function test, and a global cognitive measure. (Ref. 26) How will ADCS-PACC perform in the A4 trial?

In 2014, the A4 trial (first to attempt AD-P) proceeded with a design criterion that limited selection to at-risk volunteers. They were either genetically identified or amyloid confirmed through PET imaging. (Ref. 26)

The AD-P trials will enable researchers to expand further the sequence of biological events into the presymptomatic stages of AD. The ADCS-PACC cognitive test will be assessed in this first clinical trial use as well as refining biomarker criteria that can best predict clinical outcome and, ultimately, aid in selecting appropriate volunteers for preclinical therapeutic intervention. (Ref. 21)

Thus, the future should better define the preclinical stage of AD to determine the factors that best predict the emergence of clinical impairment and progression to eventual AD and to find a biomarker profile that will identify individuals most likely to benefit from early intervention. (Ref. 21)

Bruce's comment: Will the future take advantage of using mathematical modeling, artificial intelligence (AI), and simulations by using the data *collected from 2001 to 2013 and beyond to guide selection of volunteers, develop signature profiles for design of clinical trials whereby 100 percent participation becomes possible.*

Did *Randall Bateman* of Washington University School of Medicine in St. Louis discover the AD biomarker's Holy Grail (a blood test for brain amyloid accumulation)? The method lowers background noise enough to reveal an average 15 percent drop in the plasma ratio of Aβ42/Aβ40 in people with brain amyloid compared to those without, said Bateman. (Ref. 43)

Bateman suggested that this blood test would serve as a quick initial screen for people in preclinical or prodromal disease phases. With the costs of mass spec analysis running about one-tenth the price of an amyloid PET scan, that could create savings for large trials, which need to screen thousands of potential participants (Ref. 43). Clinical diagnostic use of the test may be possible within a few years.

Bruce's comment: If the future proves this blood test repetitive and successful, it will rank with PiB, CRISPR/Cas9, and Alzheimer's in a Dish as major twenty-first century discoveries.

Genetics

Genetics may be the most exciting discipline in the twenty-first century medical field as well as being the most promising for disease intervention. Genetics' future appears to be gaining knowledge of genes functions, variants, and association with diseases. Expectations could include identification of new genes, understanding gene variants functions, and greater applications of CRISPR/Cas9.

An August 2016 report that updated the national plan of the National Alzheimer's Project Act (NAPA), identified the following genetic achievements that infer an optimistic future. (Ref. 53)

1. Technological advances enabling the scanning of thousands of DNA samples from volunteers both with and without

AD have revolutionized the detection of gene variants (mutations). Research teams are using these data to identify rare genetic variants and examine how changes in brain structure or function (assessed from brain images and other biomarkers) are associated with genome DNA sequences

2. Recent genetic discoveries have not only identified more genes involved in Alzheimer's, but also have helped figure out what they may do. Discovering the mechanisms involved in Alzheimer's onset and progression as well as disease-related brain cognitive changes identifies pathways that might be targeted to help stop disease or protect against it.

3. Under the leadership of Rudolph Tanzi at Boston's Massachusetts Hospital, researchers developed a new three-dimensional human neural model of AD [Ref. 41] that, for the first time, contained the two proteins (AB & Tau) that are hallmarks of AD. Because it is extraordinarily difficult to mimic the brain's complexity in standard laboratory models, they used genetic engineering to spur the growth of neural stem cells in a gel. The cells formed into three-dimensional networks with the amyloid plaques and tau tangles found in the human brain. This process took just six weeks, compared with the year it takes for plaque alone to form in a mouse model. The researchers then used this new model (called Alzheimer's in a Dish) to show that in neurons with mutations in APP and PSEN-1 genes, amyloid was overexpressed and tau phosphorylation elevated. Using beta and gamma secretase blocking the formation of amyloid plaques, extra cellular space amyloid and tau with certain drugs prevented tau tangles from forming. This finding lends support to the hypothesis that amyloid triggers the cascade of events that leads to AD. However, the model is limited in its current form as it does not include the immune system's response (microglia's) or inflammation issues. The model could be expanded to include these neuro-inflammatory or vascular components along with

immune responses in the future. The model provides new encouragement that a category of drugs called beta-secretase and gamma-secretase inhibitors might ultimately benefit patients if given early enough during the disease. The new model should encourage future efforts to test existing and novel drugs as potential therapies. (Ref. 41) This study—the disease in a dish—is a brilliant piece of in vitro experimentation. The excitement it has generated will be fully manifested if it resonates with clinical findings. (Ref. 41)

Bruce's comment: Evidence indicates the death of tau proteins, which begin in the entorhinal cortex (limbic system), correlate with AD symptoms. Also, tau pathology progresses from the limbic system to the neocortex, while amyloid pathology moves in the opposite direction. (Ref. 35) *What causes the death of tau appears to be the missing answer. Is it an amyloid cascade or something else? Should research data be collected on the entorhinal cortex during AD-P trials to determine if there is a baseline level of tau in the entorhinal cortex that is only impacted when reached by amyloid progression?*

CRISPR/Cas9

What is CRISPR/Cas9? It is a very complex genetic tool that has revolutionary potential in all areas of genetics, biology, and disease intervention. The focus here is on AD and dementia. This is a two-part tool. CRISPR (Clustered Regularly Interspaced Short Palindromic Repeats) is like a computer search engine, only more precise. Cas9 is an enzyme that acts like a scissor. CRISPR locates a mutation in DNA and then Cas9 cuts the mutation out of the DNA. (Ref.57) This simple description illustrates the application of the tool. The following descriptions provide an idea of CRISPR/Cas9's potential.

1. Mutation correction: Researchers worldwide are pursuing beneficial applications of this new tool. In China, research-

ers have obtained a stem cell from amyotrophic lateral sclerosis (ALS) patients and, in their laboratory, used CRISPR/Cas9 to locate mutations in two motor genes, remove and replace them, and then, using the human genome, compare the genes for their functionality based on the mutant DNA sequencing. They found 999 aberrant transcripts. This type of research illustrates the value of knowledge gained as well as the ability to pursue the aberrant transcripts relative to the disease pathways and their progressive neurodegeneration. This is a very simple explanation with complex, difficult details omitted. There is much to do, but the future value of CRISPR/Cas9 is unpredictable.

2. Functional pathway tracking: Another powerful application of the CRISPR/Cas9 system is based on its ability to target many genomic loci simultaneously for studying gene function on a global scale. (Ref. 33)

3. Animal models are highly valuable and have been used extensively to investigate neurological disorders and to find therapeutic targets for them. Because many neurodegenerative diseases can be caused by genetic DNA anomalies, the ability of CRISPR/Cas9 to directly target a mutation, allele, or nucleotide of a gene's DNA opens a new avenue for using this new technology to create laboratory models that explore neurodegenerative diseases. (Ref. 33)

4. Human embryonic gene editing: Using the gene-editing tool known as CRISPR/Cas9, Chinese researchers have successfully edited disease-causing mutations out of viable human embryos. The embryos were created in the laboratory using eggs and sperm with mutations left over from *in vitro fertilization* treatments. In theory, the embryos could develop into a baby if implanted into a woman's uterus. Researchers in Sweden and England are also conducting gene-editing experiments on viable human embryos, but those groups have not yet reported results.

5. CRISPR/Cas9 editing: The value of this tool is the creative use of its capability. Such capability is in the application of

the Cas9 enzyme application. An example is an application not to use as a scissor that cuts a mutation but to change the mutation by modifying the chemical properties of a nucleotide, making an A to a C, etc.
6. Germline editing: Altering embryos, eggs, and sperm or their precursors is known but probably will not be the first way CRISPR/Cas9 is used to tackle genetic diseases. Doctors are already planning experiments to edit genes in body cells of patients. Those experiments come with fewer ethical questions but have their own hurdles. (Ref. 33)

CRISPR/Cas9 may be the most revolutionary tool for preventing, delaying, or curing AD in the twenty-first century. Changing an ApoE4 allele to an ApoE2 or 3 would be great. However, many questions need answers, both scientifically and ethically. Ethical concerns seem to focus on concerns with natural selection and off-target transcripts. Off-target transcripts are mutations introduced during the CRISPR/Cas9 process. The Chinese ALS article (Ref. 50) showed almost no off-target transcripts.

Genetics appear to offer many future expectations. Some of these might be the following:

1. Expect new genes to be discovered.
2. Expect functions and mechanisms of some genes to be understood and associated with brain areas and cognitive symptoms.
3. Expect the amyloid cascade hypothesis to be confirmed.
4. Expect the mechanism of amyloid's link to tau to be found and confirmed.
5. Expect Alzheimer's in a Dish to discover the AD progression mechanism and offer hope to halt the disease for symptomatic patients. Also, expect the progression mechanism to be the source for a predictive biomarker.
6. Expect CRISPR/Cas9 to become the tool to correct risk genes' isoforms and mutations in patients. (FDA has

approved Novartis's Kymriah and Gilead Science's Yescarta for certain blood cancer disease.)
7. Expect objections by advocacy groups against genetic advances that will delay progress.

Lifestyle

Once AD symptoms appear, lifestyle becomes a major player in the neurodegeneration progress. So, what does the future hold? Awareness of the benefits of exercise, diet, and continued education will hopefully achieve public acceptance like cigarettes and smoking in the twentieth century became taboo and awareness reduced use.

With people living longer, continuously challenging the brain becomes an important lifestyle need. Replace the word *retirement* with "the rewarding years." Seniors should pursue new activities, hobbies, travel, education (learn about your health, body, and brain). This book is a good start.

Normal Aging

In 1906, when AD was named, the normal lifespan was fifty years. One hundred years later, a newborn can expect to live for over one hundred years, unless there is a major catastrophic event. A longer life implies that twenty-five to thirty-five percent of it will be in "the rewarding years."

How will your body and brain perform during these years? There is no correct answer to the question as no one knows. Some behaviors provide greater chances to slow normal aging than others as indicated in the lifestyles described above. The best environmental intervention for increased lifespan in organisms is *caloric restrictions*, a strategy unlikely to be acceptable to most people. (Ref. 32)

So, what is normal? Evidence indicates that expectations during "the rewarding years" will include loss of neurons and pathways in the brain along with structural changes. The brain will shrink and lose weight. Many brain functions will decline, affecting body functions. Some examples are the following: Motor functions decline. Posture is less erect. Gait is slower, and stride length is shorter. Postural reflexes are sluggish, making individuals more susceptible to loss of balance. Muscles weakens, and bones become brittle. People sleep less and wake more frequently. Memory and problem-solving abilities begin to decline. (Ref. 32) People in their seventies and eighties recognize these changes. The key issue is to delay them if possible.

Due to age or brain diseases such as AD, people may not produce enough brain cell energy to remain fully functional. Scientists using a new mouse model discovered that an enzyme, SIRT3, might protect brain cells against stresses believed to contribute to cell energy loss. They also found that *physical exercise* increased the expression of SIRT3 (found in mitochondria, the cell's powerhouse) which helped to protect the brain against degeneration in the mice. The findings suggest that bolstering mitochondrial function and stress resistance by increasing SIRT3 levels may offer a promising therapeutic target for protecting against age-related cognitive decline and brain diseases such as AD. Exercise keeps brain cells healthy.

Evidence has shown that patients with a variant (KL-VS) of the longevity gene *klotho* have higher blood levels of the *Klotho* protein along with improved brain skills such as thinking, learning, and memory. Additional animal studies showed higher-than-normal brain levels of a receptor for the neurotransmitter glutamate, enhances cognitive function. The study suggests that drugs targeting the klotho protein could improve cognition in people at risk for AD. Expect future research efforts to incorporate and build on these advances.

Evidence leads to the fact that excessive amyloid may begin as early as twenty years before symptoms appear. Researchers have the tools (MRIs, PET scans, and CSF) to make an early identification along with monitoring progression. The research community has also developed methodologies for identifying and tracking risk volunteers. Do people with generational risks want to volunteer at age fifty or just hope for a normal life?

Bruce's comment: Develop a habit of exercising fourteen hours per week, starting at age fifty or before; follow the Mediterranean diet; decrease caloric intake; eat less; avoid brunches, salad bars, and buffets; and stimulate your brain with new lifestyle activities.

Caregiving

What does the future hold for AD patients and caregivers? The 2011 strategic change to focus research on delay and prevention, realistically segmented AD into two groups. The presymptomatic group (AD-P), assumed to be patient ages forty-five to seventy, can hope and pray for an intervention to delay the disease. *The presymptomatic group will not need caregivers,* except to satisfy stoic clinical trial protocols. The symptomatic group (AD-C), age sixty-five and up, faces the reality that there currently is no intervention for delay or cure.

Caregiving for symptomatic patient: The future for patients and caregivers of the symptomatic AD-C class is the reality that neurodegeneration will slowly continue. As indicated earlier in this book, an enjoyable life is possible for many years until the severe stage. Then, many social-economic issues magnify. During the severe stage, wandering, personal care, agitation, and anxiety become full-time patient care needs. How these needs are met presents the twenty-first century *medical dilemma.* For families who can afford the cost, there are care facilities or in-home care services. For patients who cannot afford the cost, the demands become overwhelming. Whether caregiving is the responsibility of a family, husband or wife, care organization, or government through the Secretary of Health and Human Services, challenges are everywhere. Patient care issues become major decisions with little experience on which to make the decision as well as the appropriate time to reach out for help. Issues involve a family's health and/or finances situations, quality of care facilities, quality of home health personnel, Medicare and Medicaid coverage, patient/caregiver diversity and education as well as patient/caregiver's lifestyle in planning for aging.

Some observations from Bruce's experience in caring for Ethel:

1. *Timing: Time for help is when wandering starts, when daily demands become such that patients need constant attention to maintain their interest, and/or when patients' demands cause safety issues (locking the bathroom door, cooking during the middle of the night, etc.)*
2. *Home health care (HHC): Chapter 3 identified a summary of Nevada's regulation. In the future, Nevada and all similar states should differentiate between normal aging, AD, and dementia care. HHC organizations need a doctor's order, so they can charge Medicare and Medicaid, which appears to be their lifeline and a customer's attraction. As the future AD and Dementia population increases, the demand for home health care will increase. The challenge, now and in the future, is the trade-off between home care and institutional care. Will these industries have a sufficient quality as businesses and staff to meet the demands? (See Bruce's ideas in "outside the box" below.)*
3. *AD-ADRD: Awareness of AD has increased, and related dementia is gaining attention. But addressing the future of caregiver/patient issue is at its infancy. So, what is needed?*
    a) *Education and training for HHC and institutional care services should differentiate between nonmental physical patients and dementia mental patients (body issues vs brain issues). This education and training should be for all disciplines involved with care services (from hospital personnel, doctors, and nurses to the non-medical personal care aide).*
    b) *Leadership by the secretary of Health and Human Services and secretary of education need to address these problems and issues, cause awareness, and initiate solutions. (See "outside the box" ideas below.)*
4. *Legal: Congress should provide leadership for the "outside the box" ideas suggested later in this chapter. States should address dementia as a statute separate from assisted living.*

5. *Memory Care Facility: Similar to HHC, staff makes a difference.*

    Ethel is in the Ronald Reagan Memory Support Suites (RRMSS), which is a part of Las Ventanas Continuing Care Community. This has been beneficial both economically and for staffing. According to the laws of Nevada, memory facilities are a branch under assisted living (AL) which guides the operation and staffing requirements. RRMSS has sixteen individual apartments, along with a kitchen, living area, game room, and an outside courtyard. RRMSS is a secure building which is separate from but connected to AL building. RRMSS does not staff a RN since that requirement is covered through AL staff (Bruce views this state guided requirement a detriment). The staff includes a manager, licensed nurse practitioners (LNPs), a cook, an activity director, and "Best Friends" who provide care maintenance. Service is 24/7. RRMSS size creates a family social environment that has stimulated patient-to-patient interaction where possible. Patients cover the spectrum in both age and disease. RRMSS is a high-end facility. Future patient demand is expected to far exceed the supply of available facilities. Bruce offers some ideas in Outside the Box later in this chapter for addressing future demand. Families with economic and health problems, who are burdened with AD and other dementias, pose a significant societal problem that compounds caregiving issues. These situations appear to fall to the government and/or charitable organizations.

6. *AD-P: Candidates without symptoms but either with or without amyloid (age forty-five to sixty-five) are normally functioning people and do not need caregivers. Ethel retired in January 1993 at the age of fifty-five. Later, she reflected that she had memory problems (mainly names) at that time but disregarded them because she was functioning normally. It wasn't until 2005 that her MMSE score dropped below 30. Was Ethel in a presymptomatic state for twelve years? Existing cognitive tests application have questionable use for presymptomatic patients.*

Will amyloid and tau PET scan tracers or CSF computerized fluid analysis be sufficient for determining efficacy?

Governance

What is governance? Governance is a word that can be applied very broadly to population groups in a variety of forms such as countries, states, businesses, organizations, institutions, tribes, families, etc. It relates to the processes of interaction and decision making among the stakeholders involved in a collective problem that lead to the solution of the problem or creation, reinforcement, or reproduction of norms, values, laws, and institutions.

For applying governance to Alzheimer's disease and this book, it comes down to the United States government and the stakeholders involved with dementia. More specifically, it involves Congress, the executive branch (mainly HHS) along with the medical industry and the portion of the population affected by dementia.

It wasn't until the second decade of the twenty-first century that the U.S. government passed a law that recognized AD and related (ADRD) and applied an integrated strategy of governance to a serious expanding medical issue—dementia.

Top down leadership was a key to the success in World War I and II along with the Apollo program of landing men on the moon and safely returning them to earth. These were examples of national efforts of governance that proved successful. Private contributors have mark the industrial age with leadership and inventions from the telephone to the internet. Medical science has contributed tremendously from penicillin to the human genome. So, where does that leave Alzheimer disease going into the future?

In 2009, ex-supreme court justice Sandra Day O'Conner and ex-speaker of the House, Newt Gingrich testified before Congress for a project dedicated to Alzheimer disease (AD) research. This led to the National Alzheimer's Project Act (NAPA)

Would a national strategy follow the successful results of the Apollo program organizational structure and establish a dedicated agency to guide AD research and development? This was not to be. With congressional modification of the original concept, promoted by O'Conner and Gingrich, NAPA redefine the term Alzheimer's disease to mean Alzheimer's disease and related dementia (ADRD) and designated the secretary of Health and Human Services (HHS) with responsibility to develop and implement a strategic plan to achieve a primary goal "to treat or prevent Alzheimer's disease by 2025," when NAPA terminates.

With an expansion to include related dementia, NAPA directed HHS to create an advisory council to coordinate efforts across all federal agencies and develop an Alzheimer's disease and related dementia (ADRD) plan. In May 2012, a national Alzheimer's disease and related dementia plan was released.

What is the National Alzheimer's Project Act? (NAPA)

The National Alzheimer's Project Act (Public Law 111-375), passed unanimously by Congress in December 2010 and signed into law by President Barack Obama in January 2011. (Ref. 59)

NAPA Discussion

Along with NAPA becoming law in 2011, an AD paradigm shift may have been the best decision thus far in the twenty-first century, though creating uncertainties. The uncertainties need time to be resolved. Some of these are the following:

1. Will AD presymptomatic candidates want to find out whether they possibly are on the path to AD twenty years before symptoms appear (like about age fifty)?
2. Will pharmaceutical companies invest in trials for ten to twenty years to find out whether an intervention is viable or not?

3. With the A4 clinical trial being a private/public funded effort, how will that work financially if successful?
4. With the A4 clinical trial criteria requiring open data results including volunteers, how will this work out regarding pharmaceuticals, volunteers, legal, and political issues?
5. Will the A4 selection criteria prove "not early enough" "or too early" in the disease process to determine efficacy for delay and/or prevention?
6. Are new biomarkers needed to accurately measure the unknown rate of progression changes twenty years before symptoms appear?
7. Does identification of presymptomatic AD represent a pre-existing medical condition for insurance purposes in the case of a fifty- to sixty-year-old?
8. Are new laws needed for presymptomatic trial efficacy?

These were some of the issues facing the National Alzheimer's Project Act (NAPA) advisory council in planning for innovated solutions. Congress, in writing NAPA, escalated the council issues by changing from just AD to include all related dementia (ADRD). Congress also specify the stakeholders for the advisory council that led to the structural approach for addressing the issues that were not just AD prevention or cure, but also included other dementia (ADRD), care support, agency resource centers, public/private partnerships, and epidemiology.

Despite this advocacy/lobbyist structure that encompass all possible stakeholders, some significant basic and translational research has been accomplish along with promotional awareness. It may not be the optimum for achieving goals, but it will advance knowledge that is desperately needed.

Bruce's experience in government sponsor Breeder Reactor research in the 1980s in which there was a similar advocacy structure found that organizations competed, and stronger advocates gain more funding. This diminished achieving a single objective goal.

Since dementia and the brain are both very complex and increase knowledge is needed, the current NAPA structure may be beneficial if expectations of the general population are set realistically.

Recognizing that basic and transitional research discoveries still need proof of concept via clinical trials establishes a realism that such discoveries are not near-term benefits for AD patients. It appears that the advisory council has recognized this by addressing many issues in hope of basic and translational research discoveries. These issues are reflected in the NAPA milestones that have been established and are being completed. (Ref. 38) The following selected issues provide some encouragement for the long range:

1. Modeling: Integrating mathematics with molecular biology, genetics, and AD clinical trial data, along with the advances in computer technology to accommodate big data, genetics, and laboratory experiments has created opportunities to target challenges such as
    (a) reducing the time for proof of concept via clinical trials. (Ref. 62)
    (b) creating "omics" (combination pf proteins, genetic, and molecular processing) models to study brain networks. These would include artificial intelligence's (AI) self-learning techniques. (Ref. 62)
    (c) Using modeling and longitudinal data collected for decades, develop profiles for amyloid progression along with tauopathy as well as mathematics, omics, genetics, and AI for prodromal AD extrapolations. This could possibly become a benchmark for the pre-symptomatic trials and hopefully later for eliminating the need for a placebo cohort group.
    (d) The resource section of the NAPA structure is using its funding to integrate the many data centers involved with AD and ADRD into a central system that provides secure access to any researcher. This may be an unappreciated benefit, except for the creative mind. (Ref. 62)

(e) The A4 clinical trial is a public/private partnership between the government and Eli Lilly testing Solanezumab in presymptomatic volunteers that has a completion targeted for 2022. (Ref. 61)

There appear to be issues created by AD-P that may lack visibility or recognition such as the following:

(a) *The following is from Reference 20*
  1. Current Food and Drug Administration (FDA) regulatory guidelines for AD require that *a drug show benefit for patients with AD dementia on cognition* and that clinical benefit be demonstrated either by global or staging assessment or in activities of daily living (ADL). Without symptoms, how are cognitive benefits determined? Is a new FDA regulation needed for AD-P?
  2. The trials that tested cholinesterase inhibitors for mild cognitive impairment used the onset of AD dementia as the primary outcome supported by required improvement on a cognitive test (Raschetti et al., 2007). If such cognitive and functional measures are required in the design of primary or secondary prevention trials, they will likely require nearly 10 or more years to conduct. To adequately power such a study will be challenging and add significant and possibly insurmountable costs.
  3. From a regulatory point of view, a primary prevention trial would be done to support an indication or label such as drug X is indicated for the treatment of patients at risk for AD (or have preclinical AD) to delay the onset of prodromal AD or attenuate the course of cognitive impairment. Such an indication would break new ground as it would define an at-risk state, defined by biomarkers and outcomes that fall short of currently recognized clinical states or diagnoses such as AD dementia. This requires, however, that

the at-risk state or marker be recognized as defining the target population for the drug and that the outcomes of cognitive change or onset of a subtle clinical state such as mild cognitive impairment be accepted as legitimate outcomes by regulators.

4. For early phase prevention trials, changes in the non-clinical endpoints can be reasonably accepted if the change is predictive of a clinical outcome. For AD, however, this would require demonstration that, for example, reductions in brain amyloid tracer due to an experimental drug are associated with subsequent attenuation of cognitive decline or improved quality of life. At present, it is uncertain whether current AD biomarkers can be used as surrogates for clinical measures. Indeed, at this point the field is trapped by a conundrum, we would like to use biomarkers as surrogates in clinical trials, but we have yet to establish the link between the surrogate marker with cognitive or functional endpoints.

5. The nonmedical challenges that may prove more difficult to overcome are those regarding the financial underpinnings of prevention or early intervention trials. At present there is no clear road map regarding how such trials might be financially underwritten and who receives the financial rewards if a therapy is shown to have benefit. Moreover, if the scientific and medical advances result in trial designs that are substantially more expensive, rather than less expensive, then the financial obstacles will become greater. Because there is no clear path forward at this time, a fourth step is to make certain the issues of "Who pays? and "Who gets rewarded?" are openly discussed. Indeed, all the stake holders need to recognize that this may be a critical issue to address, not only for AD prevention trials, but also prevention trials for many neurodegenerative conditions. Ultimately, addressing this obstacle may

require revisiting patent law and laws or guidelines regarding market exclusivity.

(b) *The following is from Reference 19*

The Centers for Medicare & Medicaid Services (CMS) has determined that the evidence is insufficient to conclude that the use of positron emission tomography (PET) amyloid-beta (Aβ) imaging is reasonable and necessary for the diagnosis or treatment of illness or injury or to improve the functioning of a malformed body member for Medicare beneficiaries with dementia or neurodegenerative disease, and thus PET Aβ imaging is not covered under §1862(a)(1)(A) of the Social Security Act (the Act).

However, there is sufficient evidence that the use of PET Aβ imaging is promising in two scenarios: (1) to exclude Alzheimer's disease (AD) in narrowly defined and clinically difficult differential diagnoses such as AD versus frontotemporal dementia (FTD) and (2) to enrich clinical trials seeking better treatments or prevention strategies for AD by allowing for selection of patients based on biological as well as clinical and epidemiological factors.

Therefore, we will cover one PET Aβ scan per patient through coverage with evidence development (CED) under §1862(a)(1)(E) of the Act in clinical studies that meet the criteria in each of the paragraphs below.

Clinical study objectives must be to (1) develop better treatments or prevention strategies for AD or as a strategy to identify subpopulations at risk for developing AD or (2) resolve clinically difficult differential diagnoses (e.g., frontotemporal dementia [FTD] versus AD), where the use of PET Aβ imaging appears to improve health outcomes. These may include short-term outcomes related to changes in management as well as longer term dementia outcomes.

Clinical studies must be approved by CMS, involve subjects from appropriate populations, and be comparative and longitudinal. Where appropriate, studies should be prospective, randomized, and use postmortem diagnosis as the endpoint. Radiopharmaceuticals used in the PET Aβ scans must be FDA approved.

(c) If the A4 trial was successful and approved in 2023, how would the general population candidates (age fifty to sixty-five) afford the cost (PET scan and tracers, CSF, and MRIs) of being diagnosed with presymptomatic conditions? Would such diagnosis be a pre-existing condition for insurance? Would there be insurance coverage available?

(d) Evidence $_{(Ref. 39)}$ suggests that AD symptoms start when the entorhinal cortex experiences of cell death cause by hyperphosphorylation of tau. Other evidence suggest that amyloid plaque is a trigger for the tau demise. A baseline status and tracking of the entorhinal cortex through PET scans using both amyloid and tau tracers would seem beneficial for data collection that could factor into modeling.

Bruce's comments: NAPA governance appears to be complying with the intent of NAPA as imposed by Congress and confirmed by President Obama signing it into law. A separate dedicated concept (like NASA for Apollo and beyond) as created by President Kennedy may have changed the NAPA advocacy/lobbyist structure created by Congress to a structure with an initial focus on AD and longer range plans for other dementias. However, it didn't, so between NIH and the NAPA advisory council significant basic and translational research is being accomplished along with innovative concept to use technology and state-of-the-art science applications. For anyone with motivation and time, reference 53, 59, 61, 62, and 38 provide a wealth of information.

Reality Predictions

1. The human brain is so complex that to achieve a cure for AD or even prevent or delay it will take a miracle (to use religious terms). The efficient manipulation of genetics and biology is easily achieved by the human brain, but a hor-

rendous nightmare for researchers (with all due respect). Patients and caregivers should be grateful if delaying the disease is achieved by 2033.
2. AD and dementia are not high priorities relative to the United States's social environment and the vast welfare demands. Look for solutions to come from countries other than the United States—unless there are major policy changes which are unlikely.
3. The presymptomatic strategy offers viable hope for delay. If removing amyloid and preventing plaque is confirmed to delay the damage caused by tau, then candidates with risk factors will pursue early diagnosis. This will be a major step, perhaps by 2025.
4. Most of the Baby Boomer generation will face the reality that the delay option is too late to benefit them. Generation X will have to be aware of the research outcomes, whereby their early actions could allow them to delay the disease.
5. Clinical trials will continue the placebo benchmarks, unless the science and technology for modeling develop signature AD profiles.
6. Beta amyloid vaccine (AN-1792), along with beta and gamma secretase inhibitors, will be redeemed as the right interventions but previously just targeted the wrong stages of the disease.
7. Genome sequencing, CRISPR/Cas9, PET scan tracers (nuclear medicine), and Alzheimer's in a Dish will provide tools for researchers to discover gene functions and mechanisms. This will start a new industry of medical apps (like computer apps) targeting different diseases as a part of personalized medicine.
8. By the end of the twenty-first century, researchers will gain additional significant knowledge of the brain's immune system, biomarkers, genetics, molecular biology, mitochondria, and related dementia subcategories.
9. A DNA editing apps industry will evolve that competes with chemical drugs for resolving genetic disease problems.

This will use tools like CRISPR/Cas9 and AD in a Dish to creatively develop apps (like a drug) to correct DNA variants.
10. The lack of strict and selected immigration laws and the monumental influx of illegal immigrants over the last forty years will escalate the medical dilemma for dementia during the second half of the twenty-first century in the USA.

Thinking "Outside the Box"

1. Eliminate placebo groups from clinical trials and have everyone receive the trial drug. The reference benchmark would be a mathematically developed algorithm that provides various signatures of the disease progression.
2. As lifespans continue to increase, the need for geriatric physicians will be more demanding. Through government leadership, both federal and state programs should be developed for geriatric medical students with educational incentives. Such an incentive could be a geriatric service bill (GSB) either like the GI Bill or like the armed service academies, where a free education would be provided but, upon graduation, require a year of service for each year of schooling. The graduates could then be assigned to a state-supported, diverse, low-income population, thereby providing additional caregivers where most needed. This GSB could be for doctors, nurses, and dementia memory care specialists.
3. An alternate GSB program could be an educational opportunity like the military academies. Senators and congressmen could nominate students (number to be determined). Those graduates would return to their home states to fulfill their commitments. Such a program should provide opportunities for diverse, low-income groups to advance in society.

4. Develop state-directed, diverse, low-income dementia memory communities. These could be state-run or licensed to nonprofit organizations. The facilities would employ committed graduates from the GSB program. Each state would create its own program structure (maybe like the VA or the Dept. of Motor Vehicles).
5. This GSB concept would stimulate future planning to accommodate the expected growth in the senior population and expected dementia demands in the second half of the twenty-first century.
6. Funding source ideas for the above could be (a) reduced welfare demands for diverse, low-income groups taking advantage of GSB opportunities, (b) a $0.0001 tax on all entertainment events, (c) a $0.0001 tax on all stock shares transactions (10,000-share transaction would produce one dollar), or (d) all these.

Like the thinking expressed in the Global Alzheimer's Platform (GAP) Foundation, establish dementia campuses throughout the United States (and even the world) whereby care could be provided for patients unable to support themselves. These campuses could be refurbished obsolete government facilities such as old military bases or federal buildings. The campus could be segmented by buildings or floors, each identified by dementia subcategories (AD, DLB, FTD, VD, and MID). Also, the campus concept could be promoted for philanthropic legacies.

8

Understanding Alzheimer's Disease

The key to understanding Alzheimer's disease (AD) is accepting the reality of "what is" and pursuing knowledge to manage realistic expectations that include the following:

1. There is no cure for AD as of 2017 and probably not during the first half of the twenty-first century.
2. The longer you live, the higher is the risk for late onset AD (LOAD→ +sixty-five years) which is the largest percentage of AD patients.
3. A small percentage of people inherit early onset AD (EOAD→ +thirty-five years) due to mutations in genes (amyloid precursor protein [APP], Presenilin 1 and 2 [PS1 & PS2]). Generations of people with these mutations are classified as autosomal dominant Alzheimer's disease (ASAD).
4. AD is a slow progressive disease that usually does not affect lifestyle until the severe stage (MMSE score below 10).
5. Research posits that AD begins ten to twenty years before symptoms appear.
6. Once symptoms appear, intervention is unlikely to be effective. (Refs. 16 & 39)

7. The Genetic Information Nondiscrimination Act (GINA) does not protect AD patients, whereby they could purchase life and long-term care insurance. (Ref. 42) In addition, patients could be exposed to reimbursement denials from insurers, Medicare and Medicaid.
8. Center for Medical Services (CMS) denied covering the cost of PET scan radioisotope tracers. (Ref. 19) Insurers are sure to follow this denial, which affects patients/caregiver decision-making.
9. CRISPR/Cas9 has the capability to attain delay prevention and/or cure. However, it is currently in basic and transitional research and needs additional laboratory evaluation, which is occurring. Since the capability is vast, so will be the time until it provides benefits for AD.
10. CRISPR/Cas9 potential is so great that a new genetic medical segment could evolve by the second half of the twenty-first century. It could be a future major tool in personalized medicine.
11. Genetics has the potential to correct hierarchical mutations in an embryonic stage. Will such capability be publicly accepted?
12. An AD tsunami is building. Will Bruce's "outside the box" geriatric care suggestion be heeded?

Managing realistic AD expectations include the following:

1. Enjoy the years of normal lifestyle (up to the severe stage).
2. Family/caregivers need to accept behavior changes as part of the disease and not their loved one (*always answer their questions*).
3. Caregivers should increase their knowledge of AD whereby they can anticipate decline and recognize symptoms.
4. Monitor research, clinical trials, and governance for realistic research accomplishments and expectations (see Appendix B—Websites including Bruce's www.alzheimersabc.com).

5. Follow near term AD research (2018—2025) for results from autosomal, prodromal and asymptomatic trials.
6. Follow long-term research (next twenty-five years) for progress and advances in genomics, proteomics, modeling, laboratory use of CRISPR/Cas9, new radioisotope tracers for tracking disease pathways, Alzheimer's in a Dish modeling, results of big data analysis, and understanding the brain's immune functions and mechanisms.
7. Follow medical technology advances. These might include med apps, modeling with artificial intelligence, use of virtual machines for personalized medicine, and blood test for diagnosing AD.

AD vs. Dementia

AD is one of the subcategories of dementia. Prior to 1906, senile dementia defined mental disease and memory loss. Through an autopsy, Dr. Alois Alzheimer identified a sticky substance (later called amyloid plaque) and tangles (later associated with the tau protein) as contributing to AD. Demented patients' death certificates in the twentieth century identified senile dementia as cause of death. Today, due to technology and research, PET scan tracers identify AD's plaque and tangles in vivo (living patients).

As indicated throughout this book, AD and dementia are very complex to describe and explain. The knowledge gained in the twentieth century appears overwhelming but may have only scratched the surface. Even though AD is the primary form of dementia, other dementias have been and possibly will continue to be identified as people continue to increase in age. Other identified dementias include vascular disease dementia (VDD), Lewy body dementia (LBD), frontotemporal dementia (FTD), mixed dementia, and others. Lewy body dementia includes dementia with Lewy bodies (DLB) and Parkinson's disease dementia (PDD). DLB begins with Lewy bodies in the synapse terminal, followed later by PDD motor symptoms. PDD starts with motor symptoms followed later with DLB symptoms.

The differences in each of these dementias are in symptoms, behaviors, proteins, mutations as well as areas of the brain. As these diseases progress and patients age, mixed dementia may occur. This has become common in DLB and PDD, AD and VDD, AD and DLB.

Vascular disease dementia involves cerebral amyloid angioplasty (CAA), ischemic strokes, transient ischemic strokes, and/or silent strokes. CAA is amyloid plaque buildup in the brain's arteries and veins. VDD patients may not lose memory but have symptoms associated with other brain functions that are impacted.

Lewy bodies are abnormal deposits of the alpha-synuclein protein found in the synapse terminal. DLB symptoms involve thinking, movement, behavior, visual hallucinations, sleep disorders, and mood. PDD occurs with damage to or death of dopaminergic neurons in the substantia nigra area. Cause of dopaminergic neuron demise is unknown. Symptoms are tremors, rigidity, slow movement, and postural instability.

Frontotemporal dementia main suspect is a mutation in the tau protein. Symptoms are aphasia (language disorder), behavior, and atrophy of the frontal and temporal lobes.

It is becoming common to see mixed dementia patients with AD and vascular disease dementia, AD and dementia with Lewy bodies or Parkinson's and AD. This is making the caregiving role more challenging and complex.

Loss of memory is a hallmark of AD. The loss of memory starts in the entorhinal cortex (EC). [Ref. 39] The EC functions like a computer server. As symptoms appear, damage to the EC prevents information transfer to the hippocampus for short-term memory storage and later assignment of information to long-term memory storage. Also, transfer to and from the neocortex and cerebellum become impacted. [Ref. 16] Currently, damage to the EC becomes the point of no return for AD. If the brain's immune system or drug intervention were able to prevent damage to the EC, the devastating effects of AD might not occur. However, the disease is currently not preventable, and it then attacks other areas of the brain. The neocortex, which is the last area to develop, becomes the target, where the executive functions of knowledge, learning, communication, and self are lost. At this point, the real impact of the disease becomes apparent. This was Ethel's condition at the end of 2015 with a MMSE score of 6. However, it does not stop there but proceeds to the limbic system where personality, fear, worry, anger, and insecurity begin, leading to depression, wandering, confusion, anxiety, agitation, frustration, and psychological issues. This is how Ethel began 2016 and required antidepression medication. Ethel's neurologist prescribed 15 mg Mirtazapine twice a day. Twice a day was too much as Ethel became aggressive. Reducing it to once a day proved just right. Awareness of symptoms from drug overdose is another reason for caregivers to seek knowledge.

AD Types

The paradigm shift in 2011 modified AD into two classifications: presymptomatic and symptomatic AD. Presymptomatic has two subclasses. AD Positive (AD-P) is a subclass of nonsymptomatic patients with amyloid identified by PET scan tracers or MCI above MMSE 25. Asymptomatic is the other subclass, whose patients are without amyloid, but may have heredity risk factors. The symptomatic class is AD confirmed (AD-C) where cognitive symptoms have been determined.

Prior to 2011, AD was either early onset AD (EOAD) or late onset AD (LOAD). A group of EOAD patients who inherited a mutation in their APP, PS1, or PS2 genes was identified by ADAD if their history was three generations or familial AD (FAD) if two generations. EOAD patients' symptoms appeared near age thirty-five.

The medical profession uses a language of its own, which complicates learning about and understanding AD for patients and caregiver. There are many terms that define the various risk factors or conditions by which patients develop AD. (Appendix A provides definition help.)

As indicated above, familial AD (FAD) refers to a genetic inheritance from a parent. In addition to APP, PS 1, and PS 2 for EOAD, the ApoE gene allele 4 is a high risk for LOAD. ApoE gene has an allele option of E2, E3, or E4. If the father has E2/E3 and the mother has E3/E4, then the embryo possibilities are E2/E3, E2/E4, E3/E3, or E3/E4. Therefore, a 50 percent chance of E4 is possible. If the embryo receives E2-E4, then it becomes a question of which allele is dominant? If E2 is dominant over E4, AD may not occur even with the E4 risk allele. However, if the E4 is dominate, then risks of AD increase. For the embryo with E2/E4 where the E4 is not dominant, that E4 allele still could pass to the next generation, where it could become dominant.

The amyloid precursor protein (APP) gene's mutation causes an excess of the beta amyloid peptides ($AB_{40, 42}$). Patients with this gene mutation are ADAD since amyloid is hypothesized to cascade the pathology of AD.

The largest number of AD patients is in the LOAD classification. In this classification, patients begin to display symptoms near or over age sixty-five. Known risk factors include the E4 allele of the ApoE gene, mutations in the amyloid precursor protein (APP) gene, variations of age related issues as well as lifestyle behaviors and environment. Recently, genetics has identified additional 52 genes as risk factors, most of which are involved with the brain's immune system—most notable is TREM2 gene.

With the strategic shift to prevention/delay based on evidence that AD begins ten to twenty years prior to symptoms, a classification became necessary to identify the group of patients who could proceed to develop symptoms. Therefore, this group was classified Prodromal AD (AD-P). [Ref. 21] These AD-P candidates are prodromal AD group, an asymptomatic group, and early MCI. And they carry the hope for treatment, delay, and/or prevention.

The group of patients without symptoms, but with amyloid in their brains, is determined by tests through CSF and/or PET scans tracers. Asymptomatic AD is a group of patients identified without amyloid in the brain through CSF and PET scans tracers, but who have possible risk factors through inheritance. This group also includes volunteers without risk factors.

Mild cognitive impairment (MCI) are candidates with a MMSE score higher than 25, whether with or without amyloid.

TABLE 8.1. Paradigm Shift.

Before 2011	*After 2011*
Early Onset AD (EOAD)	Autosomal Dominant AD (ADAD)
Late Onset AD (LOAD)	Familial AD (FAD)
Sporadic AD (LOAD)	Prodromal AD (PAD)
	Asymptomatic
	Late Onset AD (LOAD)
	Sporadic AD (LOAD)

Detailing AD

In addition to AD being the major part of dementia and realizing the different types of AD, this chapter provides medical and non-medical details to gain a common-sense view of AD. By building on previous chapters, these views are discussed as (1) AD's proteins, (2) protein evidence, (3) biomarkers, (4) genetics, (5) prodromal AD, (6) clinical trials, (7) lifestyle, (8) AD research and governance, (9) caregiving, and (10) Bruce and Ethel's journey. Some information may be repeated from previous chapters to aid in understanding.

1. AD's Proteins

Sticky plaques and tangles are associated with late onset AD's two causative proteins, amyloid precursor protein and tau protein. The amyloid precursor protein (APP) is a membrane protein that is concentrated in the synapses of neurons. Its function is unknown. The tau protein facilitates the nervous system's communication. Tau protein is partially in the nucleus, while an external part is in the axon (shown in figures 6.3).

Beta amyloid peptides (AB_{40-42}) from the APP have been the primary AD research targets for the past twenty-five years. As shown in figure 2.2, an enzyme (beta secretase) initially cuts the APP protein into a polypeptide (ninety-nine amino acids). An enzyme (gamma secretase) then cuts the polypeptide to forms a peptide of between thirty-six to forty-two amino acids. Peptide AB_{40} is soluble. AB_{42} is the plaque form (Appendix A—definition of peptide and polypeptide).

Excessive accumulation of AB in the brain is due to either overproduction and/or decreased clearance of AB and/or its remnants. Excess beta amyloid becomes toxic, forming fibril tissues that aggregate in external cellular space forming plaque. Where, how, and what causes the amyloid to spread is unknown, but as it spreads, amyloid is postulated to affect the tau protein. Amyloid plaque is also found in the brain's plasma systems' arteries and veins. These histological modifications have been associated with a slowly evolving cognitive deficit and memory impairment.

Tau tangles caused by hyperphosphorylation are hallmarks of AD pathology. Picture the tau protein as a set of railroad tracks connecting two towns, where the towns are like the nucleus of the neuron and the tracks are like the tau tubes going through the axons to the synapse area. Along comes hyperphosphorylation of tau (perhaps age related or caused by AB) that produces tangles. This is like twisted railroad tracks. Tangles, internal to the tau protein's nucleus, cause neuron death. Neither the mechanism, nor how this occurs, is known. Hyperphosphorylation is postulated as the cause of tangles. Evidence, found through autopsies, has shown tangles in external cellular space of donor brains.

2. Protein Evidence

AD differs from other forms of dementia by its specific pathology, genetic risk factors, and functional stages of cognitive decline (as described for Ethel in chapter 3). AD is associated with a specific pattern of pathological changes in the brain that result in neurodegeneration (neuron's dying) and the progressive development to dementia. Pathological hallmarks common to the disease include beta-amyloid plaques, dystrophic neurites associated with plaques and neurofibrillary tangles within nerve cell bodies. The exact relationship between these pathological features has been elusive, although beta-amyloid plaques precede neurofibrillary tangles in *neocortical areas*. (Ref. 35)

Autopsy examination of the brains of some individuals in the preclinical stage of the disease have shown that the earliest form of neuronal pathology associated with beta-amyloid plaques resembles the cellular changes that follow structural injury to axons (such as in boxing or football). Likewise, the development of beta-amyloid plaques in the brain may cause physical damage to axons. Abnormally prolonged stimulation of the neuronal response may result in neurofibrillary pathology and neurodegeneration. Therapeutically, inhibiting neuronal immune response to either beta amyloid plaque or physical trauma may be useful neuroprotective strategies in the earliest stages of AD (Ref. 2) (*If injury to axons and dendrites cause pathological damage and not necessarily loss of neurons, could memory still be available but just not accessible? Could such injuries to axons and dendrites be repaired in the future?*)

AD autopsies identified damaged connections between neurons (axons and dendrites). As tangles occur internal to the cell, neurons are lost.

Decades of research's evidence has not only identified the need for more knowledge of many brains functions but strongly implicates that beta amyloid accelerates tau pathology and the neurodegeneration process leading to MCI and AD. (Ref. 58) The evidence also suggests delay and/or prevention is a possibility, if therapeutics can be successful prior to symptoms appearing. The good news is that our children and grandchildren may benefit. The bad news is that once symptoms appear, the disease has progressed past the point for effective intervention.

AD symptoms begin with memory issues. The entorhinal cortex (EC), located in the middle of the temporal lobe, plays a crucial role as a gateway connecting the neocortex and the hippocampal formation (figure 6.4). *(This gateway is the key for connecting memory to the executive functions of learning, communicating, decision making, and basic intelligence).* Autopsy analysis provides evidence that there are approximately seven million neurons in the adult human EC. (Ref. 16) No significant loss of neurons in the EC is detectable in cognitively normal subjects between the sixth and ninth decades of life. However, the EC is severely affected (~33 percent lost neurons) in very mild AD cases. (Ref. 16) The neuronal loss was so significant that it must have started well before the onset of symptoms. This led to a recommendation to develop new diagnostic tests that would predict presymptomatic AD, before massive neuronal loss occurred and when therapeutic intervention might be most effective. (Ref. 16) There is no recovery once neurons are lost. *Unfortunately, it took twenty years of technology development (mainly MRIs and PET scans) to be able to pursue this 1996 autopsy study's recommendation to develop diagnostics for presymptomatic AD*

In 1991, through autopsies of donated brains from nondemented and demented patients, Heiko Braak and Eva Braak defined a classification for stages of tau pathological progression from the entorhinal cortex to the neocortex. (Ref. 39) Twenty-five years later, with the technological development of positron emission tomography (PET) scans and a nuclear medicine tracer (AV1451), researchers duplicated the autopsy classification in vivo (living humans). (Ref 35)

AV1451 is the most widely studied tau PET tracer to date. Overall, researchers showed largely converging results indicating that tau correlates more strongly than amyloid with neurodegeneration and cognitive decline in AD. This data strengthens a growing belief that while amyloid and tau pathology first start up independently in separate regions in an aging person's brain, the presence of amyloid in a tau area somehow intensifies and accelerates an otherwise limited tauopathy. (Ref. 47) "Exactly how that happens is one of the great mysteries in AD research these days," said Reisa Sperling of Harvard Medical School. *(The Braak and Braak classification and the AV1451 classification provide strong evidence that tauopathy is limited without an amyloid promoter. Therefore, developing therapeutic intervention to treat patients long before symptoms appear supports the current strategy of delay and/or prevention.*

Evidence has shown, that once symptoms appear, clearance of amyloid plaque does not prevent the disease from continuing. (Ref. 18) Evidence also indicates that tau tangles correlate with cognitive symptoms and decline. (Ref. 58) Though evidence indicates a relationship between amyloid and tau, the connecting link is elusive. (Ref. 58)

3. Biomarkers

Chapter 6 described the two classes of AD biomarkers (clinical and cognitive). Chapter 7 described biomarkers' future along with present issues. Biomarkers are tools to measure variance against established norms like blood data does for the body and a thermometer does for temperature. Both blood analysis and thermometers are cost effective diagnostic tools. Detailing status of biomarkers for AD follows.

CSF, MRIs, and PET scans have made enormous improvements for clinical trials and research analysis but are questionable for the general population diagnosis. Many constraints limit their application like prediction of disease progression and onset, along with being costly and invasive.

Cognitive biomarker ADCS—PAAC was designed to provide sensitive measurements (very small changes) for the A4 clinical trial. Its challenges include a nonhomogeneous selection of volunteers (volunteers with various degrees of amyloid at baselines and progression during trial period), uncertain quality of subjective responses by volunteers/caregivers, confirmation of its statistical extrapolation of data from symptomatic trials and comparing cognitive progressive decline with clinical data results from CSF, PET scans, and MRIs.

Radioisotope agents will probably rank with CRISPR/Cas9 as contributing the most to AD research during the beginning of the twenty-first century. These agents have allowed researchers to investigate the brain and follow amyloid and tau pathology that was previously only possible in postmortem autopsies. These agents use nuclear isotopes with varying degrees of half-lives (for stability) and attach to amyloid and tau particles. Radiation quotas for volunteers could become a concern. This technology is in its infancy. Improvements are surfacing yearly. Thinking "outside the box," these agents could become like apps in the computer industry, where the intervention's design targets various proteins, maybe alleles, brain sections, functions of the brain, and/or possibly immune system response of glial cells. Are such agents needed as biomarkers for presymptomatic patients who are functioning normally without symptoms but with amyloid that is changing slowly with uncertain detectable change? Could this start a new niche industry? Drawbacks include radiation dose limits, cost, and government regulations. Appendix E describes current radioisotope activity.

Longer term, there are nonmedical challenges—financial and regulatory issues that may prove more difficult to overcome than those of a cost-efficient biomarker, AD prevention, or successful early intervention trials. FDA approval is currently regulated for interventions that treat patients with AD identified by cognitive symptoms or evidence of daily living decline. CMS reimbursements are currently tied to proof of benefit criteria under the Social Security Act. Without congressional change, it could likely require nearly ten or more years to conduct such prevention trials. "Who pays? Who gets rewarded?" Who provides patient insurance? Will this require revisiting patent law, and laws or guidelines regarding market exclusivity? Will any of this be resolved by 2033?

4. Genetics

While developmental research has been conducting drug trials mainly focused on beta amyloid, genetics has been making tremendous laboratory advances such as the following.

1. The human genome sequence was completed in 2003.

2. DNA sequencing technology, along with big data analysis, has identified additional AD risk genes (fifty-two and counting as of June 2017).
3. In the laboratory, skin stem cells were genetically engineered into induced pluripotent cells (embryonic progenitor cells), from which any desired body cell can be produced.
4. In the laboratory, a three-dimensional model of amyloid precursor protein and tau protein cells, Alzheimer's in a Dish, was created whereby amyloid plaque and tau tangles were analyzed.
5. In a Chinese laboratory, CRISPR/Cas9, a tool to locate and replace variants (mutations), was successfully used (with an egg and sperm from in vitro fertilization scheduled for disposal) to change mutations in an embryo.
6. Genome sequencing determined the order of three billion chemical letters in the DNA of 580 patients. (Ref. 53) This is a key strategy for identifying new clues to the fundamental cause of AD, and the development of new diagnostics and treatments.
7. Could CRISPR/Cas9 be to the medical field what the microchip invention was for technology during the second half of the twenty-century and beyond. As indicated in chapter 7, it has already received FDA approval for use in some blood cancers. Other applications in laboratory use and investigations include correcting the mutation that causes blindness, fixing a heart mutation in embryos, and creating new laboratory mice for AD.

Basic research laboratories are striving to understand how risk genes, their functions, and mechanisms influence AD. Genome DNA and RNA sequencing, along with identifying variants (mutations), provide data not only to identify risk genes but also to search for an understanding of a gene's function and mechanisms. In addition, researchers are sequencing the whole exome (see Appendix A definition) of an additional eleven thousand volunteers, including six thousand with Alzheimer's and five thousand controls. (Ref. 53)

This provides a foundation for further research targets that might affect AD and/or *increase understanding of protein production in a cell (proteomics)*.

The above advances may be just the tip of discoveries and may be why genetics could prove to be the future hope for preventing or curing AD. (Reminder: from basic laboratory research to the market is about twenty years.)

5. Prodromal Ad

The 2011 paradigm shift [Ref. 20] supported Braak and Braak's 1991 autopsy opinions [Ref. 39] that AD must start many years before symptoms appear. The strategy shift established a hypothesis that defined a period of ten to twenty years as a prodromal AD classification. Fortunately, the 2004 technology discovery of PET scan tracers (PiB) provided the tool for the identification of amyloid and tauopathy in living humans. Clinical trials can now select candidates with certainty of amyloid in their brains. However, these positive developments come with future uncertainties (see chapter 7).

With decades of clinical trial data based mainly on mild and moderate patient symptoms, presymptomatic efficacies predictions might not only have uncertainties, but may also be realistically questionable.

Autosomal and prodromal clinical trials are currently in progress with most completions targeted for the early 2020s. Uncertainties in these trials appear to be lack of predicting an expected time between a volunteer's baseline level of amyloid and appearance of symptoms along with the amyloid accumulation loads along the way, thereby measuring delay and efficacy. As of August 2017, these trials were using either monoclonal antibodies to target amyloid in volunteers known to have amyloid or volunteers with ADAD. Clinical biomarker evidence (CSF, PET scans, and MRIs) are the trials' indicators to determine if delay is occurring. Can this be determined without predicted expectation? In addition, cognitive evidence could be questionable because the amount of cognitive change may possibly be too small to provide definitive evidence. Claims of preventions appear unreasonable due to an uncertain time for symptoms to appear.

During the Alzheimer's Association International Conference that took place on July 16–20, 2017, in London, researchers proposed and discussed a primary prevention trial that would test one hundred to two hundred ADAD candidates without amyloid with a beta secretase inhibitor. The candidate selection would be from the DIAN participants' families. Selection criteria would be eighteen to twenty-four years of age (average twenty-two years before symptoms). Clinical biomarker would be PET imaging. Cognitive biomarkers were undetermined. Length of the trial would be four or five years to determine if preventing the start of amyloid occurred versus placebos. A continuation would follow to assess cognitive decline for those showing amyloid. Ethical concerns were raised due the child-bearing age of the candidates, and if pregnancies occurred, would a fetus be impacted?

Bruce's Comment: Is five years long enough to confidently confirm prevention or has delay just occurred? Would DIAN data be used as a prediction benchmark and a baseline for measurement and efficacy?

Could PET scan tracers monitor the entorhinal cortex (EC), determine the length of time for amyloid pathology to reach the EC from the neo-cortex, confirm that amyloid causes tau to accelerate, and produces cognitive impairment (MCI) symptoms? Could the mechanisms of amyloid to tau be found along the way?

6. Clinical Trials

Clinical trials are developmental research's proof of concept, if successful. Optimism, at the start of the twenty-first century, for a quick AD cure or prevention possibly created misguided judgments and unrealistic expectations.

In hindsight, developmental research, with its aggressive push for proof of concept may have been premature for the level of knowledge available from basic research and the technology available at the time. Lesson learned indicate that some trials may have selected the right therapeutic targets but tested patients at the wrong stage of the disease. (Ref. 25) In addition, the right drug may have had the right target, but the wrong dose, along with the wrong disease stage.

Table 8.2 shows some of the research advances that contributed to the paradigm shift in 2011 to redirect strategy from cure to delay and prevention as well as switching trial focus from mild and moderate stage patients to those with presymptomatic conditions and MCI. This shift aligned with Braak's autopsy evidence that AD began many years before symptoms. PET scan tracers confirmed Braak's 1991 classification for stages and progression and provided capability to identify amyloid and tau in a living human through PET scan images.

Table 8.2

2000 to 2017 Significant Advancement	*Year*
Human Genome Sequence Completed	2003
Positron Emission Topography (PET) Scan Radioisotope Tracers → Pittsburg Compound B (PiB)	2004
MRI's Advances	Ongoing
DNA Sequencing	2008
Big Data	2012
PET Scan Tracers (Amyloid)	2012
CRISPR/Cas9	2012
PET Scan Tracers (Tau)	2014
Alzheimer's in a Dish	2014
Induced Pluripotent Stem Cells (iPSC)	2014
In Vitro Fertilization Embryo Mutations Corrected by CRISPR/Cas9	2016

Clinical trials are not just for proof of concept of *new* AD drug candidates. Related diseases and repurposing existing drugs are now being considered as well as other potential nonpharmaceutical interventions. These include (1) impact of cardiovascular disease,

(2) impact of diabetes, (3) repurposing cancer drugs, (4) evaluating exercise benefits, (5) biomarkers proof of concept, (6) impact of nutrition, (7) confirmation of age-related cognitive decline, (8) determining value of home-based interventions, and (9) efficacy of cognitive training.

In addition, clinical trials are conducted relative to AD and related dementia (ADRD) symptoms. These include (1) delirium, (2) neuropsychiatric disorders, (3) depression, (4) agitation, (5) sleep apnea, and (6) apathy.

Dementia complexities are not just with the disease elements but also with the complexities associated with funding and strategic management.

7. Lifestyle

Along with the many advances in the twentieth century came an extended lifespan. Human lifespan in 1900 was fifty years. Newborns in 2000 can expect to live one hundred years or more. The prime trigger for all dementias, including AD, is age. Without cure or prevention, lifestyle may be the only logical approach to delaying AD and dementia. Ethel began her seventeenth year of AD in October 2017. Bruce believes her active, healthy lifestyle, along with a successful educational and professional career, always with a positive attitude, contributed to slowing the rate of decline.

To cite a different example, smoking was a cause of lung cancer during the twentieth century. A major awareness program reduced the number of smokers and related lung cancer victims. Perhaps an awareness of one's lifestyle may delay AD.

What is lifestyle? Lifestyle is the sum of choices made by people who are mentally capable—whether teenager, young adult, or senior citizen. Appropriate or inappropriate, lifestyle decisions are influenced by families, peers, educators, ideologies, environment, and cultures. President John F. Kennedy indirectly emphasized lifestyle choices in his 1961 inaugural address with these words: *"Ask not what your country can do for you, ask what you can do for your country."*

The point is whether you are an asset or liability. Appropriate lifestyle becomes an asset. Inappropriate lifestyle becomes a liability. Lifestyle is not a complete answer but increases the odds to slow or delay AD decline.

The human species functions through chemicals. These chemicals are from food and the environment. The brain receives its source of chemicals from blood. The blood provides oxygen, nutrients, amino acids, fats, proteins, carbohydrates, vitamins, and minerals. The choices made by a human, relevant to chemical inputs influence the functions of that human's organs, including the brain. (Example: smoking causes lung cancer.) Choices not only affect the decision maker but also may influence future generations. Past decision makers may have affected the DNA of the current decision maker. Decisions are made each day as to the chemicals that challenge the organs of the human body. These challenges include daily diets, alcohol, medical drugs, recreational drugs, and smoking, along with the amount of caloric intake. The body and brain each include an immune system to control and manage anomalies. Inappropriate chemical intake diminishes the effectiveness of the immune system's capabilities. The immune systems say, "Ask not what I can do to you, but ask what you shouldn't do to me."

Aging is a process like a bell curve (figure 8.1), where there is an increase in growth, energy, and the brain's executive function. Midlife is a period of raising a family and working where stress, pleasures, and behaviors influence organs, including

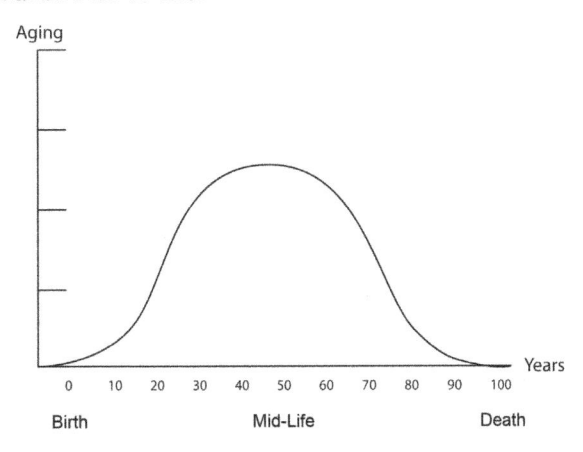

Fig. 8.1 Aging Bell Curve

the brain. As the bell curve declines, so do the organs, mainly in accordance with a chosen lifestyle. Birth → Midlife → Death

Managing lifestyle appropriately is a logical way to flatten the bell curve and slow the decline. Exercise stimulates the heart and lungs to supply oxygenated blood to the brain's neurons and immune cells. A correctly chosen diet aids in flattening or stretching the bell curve and maintaining the balance of chemicals needed for the brain's protein production. Social interaction contributes through regulation of the functions that control various organ behaviors (ego, stress, fear, fight, flight, confidence, pleasures, etc.).

Though a 2017 clinical trial did not endorse lifestyle changes to prevent AD, it did not offer an opinion on delay. The fifth edition of *Principles of Neurological Science* (PNS) (Ref. 32) states that successful aging comes through caloric restriction. PNS also indicates that people's caloric restriction is protected through childbearing years by genes and enzymes in the body's reproductive systems. However, it appears protections ends, and caloric restriction becomes each person's lifestyle responsibility. The older a person becomes, the less chemical intake is needed, if correctly selected.

Diet suggestions are (1) fats → salmon and fatty acids; (2) proteins → eggs and meats; (3) carbohydrates rice and sour dough bread; (4) vitamins A → carrots, B → nuts, C → oranges, D → sunlight and mushrooms; (5) minerals → iron → meats, sodium → salt, calcium → milk.

A 2017 to 2021 clinical trial, MIND, a three-year intervention of a hybrid of the Mediterranean and DASH diets is assessing cognitive decline among six hundred individuals who are sixty-five plus years of age, who are without cognitive impairment but are overweight and have suboptimal diets that may place them at risk for developing dementia. The MIND diet emphasizes natural, plant-based foods, limits foods that are high in animal and saturated fats and specifies green leafy vegetables and berries. Trial volunteers will be randomly assigned to eat either the MIND diet or their usual diet. Both groups will undergo mild caloric restriction for weight loss (250 calories a day) and will receive counseling to help reduce caloric intake. To assess the diet's effect on cognitive decline, researchers will measure changes in cognitive function and brain volume as well as biomarkers of oxidative stress, inflammation, and Alzheimer's disease.

A final lifestyle recommendation is to challenge not only the body, but also the brain → use it, or lose it.

Table 8.3. Lifestyle Differences.

Normal Aging	*Alzheimer's Disease*
People sixty to ninety years have no neuron loss in the transentorhinal cortex.	Alzheimer's patients have a 30 percent loss of neuron in the transentorhinal cortex when symptoms appear.
"Senior moments" are common.	"Senior moments" progress to cognitive impairment and dementia.
Many synapses in the neocortex and other brain regions decline.	Synapses become filled with amyloid plaque and neurofibrillary tangles.
Elderly brains are less able to support synchronization of complex activities due to loss of white matter in the prefrontal and temporal cortex (executive function).	AD neurodegeneration progression causes loss of neuron to recall memory and perform executive functions.

Bruce's Lifestyle Recommendations:
1) *Develop an exercise habit of "at least" thirty minutes/day from age fifty.*
2) *Avoid taking recreational drugs and, if possible and practical, medical drugs.*
3) *Consider eating like the "hunters and gathers" (five different fruits/day, five different nut groups/day, along with needed nutrients).*
4) *Reduce caloric intake with each year you age after childbearing years (~fifty years).*
5) *Maintain your health to avoid surgery and anesthesia.*

6) *Listen to your body for anomalies signals and needed rest.*
7) *Give your body and brain's immune systems the opportunity to cure anomalies.*

8. Alzheimer Disease Research and Governance

Research and awareness of AD escalated together during the 1980s. Nearly forty years later, progress is in the eye of the beholder. Beginning with analysis of autopsies and longitudinal studies, the challenges came from exploring uncharted territory. The advances in AD might parallel technology advances since landing a man on the moon in 1969. As the microchip advanced the computer industry, the identification of the APP and tau tangles identified the targets for AD research.

Braak and Braak insights provided a view of AD progression by stages of the tau protein based on autopsies' evidence. (Ref. 39) Braak's evidence included the view that the disease started many years before symptoms appeared. Braak's reported evidence identified a path forward for AD research.

Creating transgenic mice for laboratory testing during the late 1990s provided researchers a valuable tool to assess interventions. The focus was on the beta amyloid peptide and either preventing or clearing its excess remnants, including plaque. These laboratory tests guided many clinical trials to attempt intervention during the first decade of the twenty-first century.

The failed trials from 2000 through 2010 indicated the disease was too far advanced in mild and moderate stage volunteers for efficacy. The possibility that the interventions may have been conceptually correct but required an earlier stage became the strategy for the second decade of the twenty-first century.

Without having the technology advances shown in table 8.1 above, the contributions by researchers from the early 1980s to the end of 2010 are commendable.

With the technical advances shown in table 8.1, along with leadership guidance that is evolving through the National Alzheimer's

Project Act (NAPA), expectations for delay, and prevention, may be realistic during the 21st century.

However, the goal, "Prevent and efficiently treat Alzheimer's disease by 2025," in the NAPA National Plan appears ambitious and improbable. What are realistic expectations? You be the judge based on the following:

1. Presymptomatic immunotherapy trials are in progress to prevent or delay AD in MCI and Prodromal AD participants, with results expected in 2020 to 2023. Delay seems more likely as prevention may take many more years to confirm, due to the uncertain decline progression in presymptomatic stages. Chances with other related type dementias are unlikely.
2. Big data analysis models of genetic variants (mutations) are being developed and compared with trial data. These models are using artificial intelligence (AI) learning algorithms to determine pathways and disease networks. These types of innovative computer technology models may unravel complexity and identify realistic intervention targets. This is encouraging but has uncertainties as to length of time to develop and confirm such models as well as encountering unexpected complexities along the way.
3. The ability to capitalize on genomics, AD data sources, and the innovative models being developed creates a challenge to innovate placebo signature models that would allow 100 percent patient participation in trials. This would be another paradigm shift and could prove more beneficial compared to some of the current NAPA care and service recommendations.
4. The brain's immune system is just beginning to receive research attention as a possible contributor to AD. The roles of glial cells contain many unknowns. Is the immune system playing a role in tau tangles, death of neurons, and cognitive decline?

5. Genomics, sequencing, mRNAs, and proteomics are all receiving study grants. What will these studies uncover? This appears to be the right long-range strategy.
6. CRISPR/Cas9 is an infant tool that has tremendous potential. It may be the tool that unravels many mysteries through creative research applications and given sufficient time.
7. Are these too many unknowns to be pressured by the goal of 2025? It seems a realistic strategy is to continue pursuing biological and molecular understanding of the disease and take advantage of technology, modeling, and available data to unravel AD complexities.

Unknowns and uncertainties appear to make AD prevention improbable near term. However, near term expectations for delay interventions by mid-twenty-first century could be realistic based on the following:

1. Continued technology advances (like table 8.1), especially in mathematical modeling.
2. Increased strategic studies and analysis (like big data, modeling, and artificial intelligence tools).
3. Increased knowledge of "omics," namely genomics (mutations and gene networks) and proteomics (production of proteins).
4. Development of innovative applications such as PET scan tracers for network analysis (entorhinal cortex), and expansion of Alzheimer's in a Dish modeling for ApoE4, TREM2, and glial cells.
5. Promotion of a cultural paradigm shift toward a societal awareness and an investment in lifestyle behaviors, mainly exercise and diet.

9. Caregiving

Understanding caregiving for AD patients requires segmentation by classifications and disease stages. Classifications might be caregivers who can manage their own situation and those who are not capable to do so because of financial, intellectual, or diversity issues. Disease stages vary in time and onset of symptoms but mostly in a sequential pattern. AD does not know there are classifications. Caregivers often confuse other dementia or mixed dementia symptoms with AD. Chapter 7's "Thinking outside the Box" section provides ideas and suggestions of how to help those not capable of managing AD.

Caregivers capable of managing patients have two subcategories: families and institutional care. Institutional care is mostly when a patient reaches the severe stage of the disease. Whether family or institutional care, interpersonal skills, knowledge of the disease, and appropriate training are all valuable.

An AD patient begins with normal independent desires. Driving, traveling, socializing, and personal desires are all expectations. As AD progresses, doubt enters the patient's environment and a mixed period of transitioning from independence to dependence on the caregiver begins. *Me and My Shadow* depicts the patients' need for dependence and for their security. As the executive function of the neocortex loses neurons, the severe stage is reached and consideration for institutional care becomes an option.

During the independent period, caregivers need to recognize personality anomalies as symptoms and have patience, offer support, and don't become frustrated (easier said than done). Always answer questions, no matter how often asked. Respect the patients and remember they still have their egos.

During the transition stage, symptoms become more obvious and the caregiver is faced with decisions such as driving privileges, legal powers, financial controls, and end-of-life choices (personal, financial, heirs, possessions, etc.). These are all important while the patient can still communicate.

Dependence is where the caregiver interpersonal skills are valuable as patients want both independence and dependence. They also still desire to socialize, though they are losing a rational communication ability. Always provide positive support.

At the severe stage, care can become a twenty-four-hour task. At this point, either in-home care or memory care facility is needed. This decision is influenced by behavior, wandering, sundowning, bathing, toileting, etc. Recognize that transfer to a memory care facility includes an adjustment period for both the patient and caregiver and is a significant emotional event. Usually at this stage the patient has no memory recall, and everything is "at the moment." This is where redirection becomes the key tool to manage patients. After a visit to memory care, the patient doesn't remember the caregiver visited. However, the caregiver could leave with guilt feelings. Memory care personnel always used redirection. Caregiver and families also should accept and use this tool.

The following seven paragraphs are from the National Alzheimer Project Act (NAPA) FY 2019 Professional Judgment Budget submittal. (Ref. 62) A professional judgment budget is a submittal directly to the president and cannot be change by Congress.

In one recent study (Amjad et al., 2016), lack of continuity in care was linked to higher rates of hospitalization, emergency department visits, testing, and healthcare spending for fee-for-service Medicare beneficiaries.

Behavioral problems such as agitation, aggression, and apathy are common among Alzheimer's patients. They are disabling for patients and among the most troubling behaviors for caregivers.

Caregivers of people with dementia cite important emotional rewards, but many are also burdened with the significant emotional, physical, and financial toll of caregiving.

Caring for a loved one at home is particularly challenging, with additional emotional strains that can lead to caregiver fatigue, depression, and anxiety. In addition, caregivers can face economic stress from lost income and the expense of attending to someone with dementia. Eventually, families can be forced to seek institutional care, which may be more manageable, although likely more expensive, when care at home becomes too difficult to continue.

More than one million Americans have advanced dementia (Hebert et al., 2003) and experience loss of meaningful communication, total functional dependency, and a median survival rate of 1.3 years (Mitchell et al., 2009). Their families face difficult care choices on issues such as tube feeding, infections, and falls. These wrenching choices are usually made in nursing homes, often with a limited amount of time to discuss and decide.

Pneumonia, febrile (*fever*) episodes, and eating problems are frequent complications in patients with advanced dementia, and these complications are associated with high six-month mortality rates. Distressing symptoms and burdensome interventions are also common among such patients. Patients with health care proxies, who understand the prognosis and clinical course, are likely to receive less aggressive care near the end of life.

Continuity of care—consistent treatment over time by the same healthcare professional or small healthcare team—*is considered the ideal for Alzheimer's patients.*

Bruce Comments: Las Ventanas exemplifies this ideal for Alzheimer's patients, with its continual care offerings that include all levels of care and especially the Ronald Reagan Memory Support Suites. Also, knowledge and understanding of AD, as provided by this book, gives a caregiver tools to manage the journey.

10. Bruce and Ethel's AD Journey

The one thing that you want to achieve from your college education is *"the ability to apply what you learned to how you find answers and solutions to issues and problems that you encounter after graduation."* This was advice that Bruce received from his brother Raymond Bauer. This guidance has been beneficial during our AD journey.

On 9/11/2001, Bruce and Ethel found themselves at dinner in Salzburg, Austria, with Ethel's sister and brother-in-law, Joan and John Kunz. We were on a month-long vacation trip planned by Bruce.

After a week in Switzerland, a week at Lake Constance (bordering Switzerland, Austria, and Germany), a week in Austria, and concluding with a week in Munich and Oktoberfest, we came home to our paradigm shift. During Ethel's October 2001 physical, Dr. Shin informed us that she had AD. After confirming this, along with the disclosure of an ApoE 3 and an ApoE 4 allele, our difficult journey began.

Over the past seventeen years, the disease slowly progressed from a presymptomatic stage to a post severe stage. Ethel's current mental condition is about the level of a two-year old child. Though her physical condition is declining, blood tests indicate normalcy.

Ethel's personality and positive outlook have made the journey longer and better than expected. Except for a few minor issues, our lifestyle from 2001 to 2011 was not impacted. Ethel continued table tennis, computer games, social activities, and hosting dinners and parties. We continued playing golf and traveling.

As the disease became more evident in late 2011, we relocated to Las Ventanas Continuing Care facility in Las Vegas, anticipating the need for future memory care. Ethel remained active and involved from 2012 to 2016, when she transferred to the Las Ventanas Ronald Reagan Memory Support Suite. February 2018 completed two years in this facility at Las Ventanas. Bruce has lunch with her every day as she is only fifty yards away in the next building. Bruce stopped taking Ethel to the main dining room for dinner after the first year due to uncertainty of behavior occurrences. Instead, he visits Ethel after dining. The journey is ongoing.

Bruce's journey led to this book. The hardest part of the journey was, and still is seeing the person you loved, respected, admired, and enjoyed for over fifty-six years lose her exceptional mind and the ability to interact through her verbal witty personality that won everyone's love and respect, whether it was friend, family, neighbor, coworker, college roommate, or international peer.

As with most people confronted with the task of caregiving, Bruce knew nothing about AD or much about the medical field. Available published material was either extremely technical or just stories of behavioral symptoms. In addition, the medical field reports were like learning a foreign language.

Recalling the advice, he received during his college education and with the technology growth of the internet, Bruce applied those skills along with his engineering experience to pursue an understanding of AD. Researchers' answers to Bruce's e-mail questions were amazing and admirably appreciated. His knowledge of the disease accelerated when he began writing this book in 2014. In addition to this book, Bruce has written monthly articles about AD, the brain, and lifestyle for friends and residents of Las Ventanas. During 2017, he conducted classes on dementia for Las Ventanas residents and accepted an invitation to make a caregiver presentation at an Alzheimer's Foundation Association Conference held during March 2017 in Las Vegas.

Bruce has observed other forms of dementia during Ethel's residence in memory care. All patients in memory care have brain deficiencies in some area that is either from normal aging (one is 102) or a form of dementia and is observable in various behavioral issues, many of which appear worse than AD.

The journey continues and, as for the last seventeen years, you learn to play the cards you are dealt and live one day at a time as in the Doris Day song "Que Sera, Sera." (Whatever will be, will be.)

This book was written to provide a basic understanding of AD. Make it a reference guide and reread the technical parts, use the appendices and continue to increase your understanding of AD along with cementing your knowledge. Learn to anticipate the next part of the journey.

If you found this book helpful and would like to keep informed, you can go to Bruce's website — www.alzheimersabcs.com for articles and blogs. (Also, in Appendix B)

Some Parting Views

1. The human body is a chemical factory—treat it accordingly with appropriate intake and lifestyle.
2. The immune system (body and brain) provide the best care for most medical issues. Let it do its job.

3. Take responsibility for your own personal and medical decisions and consciously seek the best medical advice.
4. AD and dementia delay, prevention, and cure must be resolved through scientific knowledge and dedication of researchers—not by concerns for funding advocacy and social equality.
5. Do not just desire free medical care via Medicaid, but desire that your medical freedom is not lost to the health dictates of government.
6. AD and dementia are significant emotional diseases that require caregiver's strength, realism, and compassion for loved ones—with government care as a last choice.
7. Low income diversity is like the fishing parable. "Provide a person a fish meal and you provide one meal; teach a person how to fish and you provide them how to eat for life." Could Bruce's chapter 7 "outside the box" idea for a Geriatric Service Bill (GSB) offer low income diversity population the opportunity to learn how to fish?

References

Ref. 1:
Schenk, Dale et. al. "Immunization with Amyloid-β Attenuates Alzheimer-Disease-Like Pathology in the PDAPP Mouse." *Nature 400*. (July 8, 1999): 173–177.

Ref. 2:
Vickers JC, Dickson TC, Adlard PA, Saunders HL, King CE, McCormack G. "The Cause of Neuronal Degeneration in Alzheimer's Disease." (Feb. 2000).

Ref. 3:
Alzforum. "Human Aβ Vaccine Snagged by CNS Inflammation." (Jan. 3, 2002).

Ref. 4:
"More Cases of Brain Inflammation in Vaccine Trial." *Washington Post*. (Feb. 25, 2002).

Ref. 5:
Nicoll JA, Wilkinson D, Holmes C, Steart P, Markham H, Weller RO. "Neuropathology of Human Alzheimer's Disease after Immunization with Amyloid-Beta Peptide—a Case Report." *Nat Med*. (4) (Apr. 9, 2003):448–52.

Ref. 6:
Greenberg, S. M., B. J. Bacskai, B. T. Hyman. "Alzheimer Disease's Double-Edged Vaccine." *Nat Med.* (4) (Apr. 9, 2003):389–90.

Ref. 7:
Orgogozo, J. M., MD, S. Gilman, MD FRCP et al. "Subacute Meningoencephalitis in a Subset of Patients with AD after Aβ42 Immunization." (July 2003).

Ref. 8:
Christoph Hock et al. "Antibodies against β-Amyloid Slow Cognitive Decline in Alzheimer's Disease." 38, issue 4. (May 22, 2003): 547–554.

Ref. 9:
"Philadelphia: Can a Shrinking Brain Be Good for You?" International Conference on Alzheimer's Disease. (July 22, 2004).

Ref. 10:
Boche D[1], Donald J, Love S, Harris S, Neal JW, Holmes C, Nicoll JA. "Reduction of Aggregated Tau in Neuronal Processes but not in the Cell Bodies after Abeta42 Immunization in Alzheimer's Disease." (July 22, 2004).

Ref. 11:
S. Gilman, MD, FRCP, et.al. "Clinical effects of Aβ immunization (AN1792) in patients with AD in an interrupted trial." *Neurology* 64, no. 9 (May 10, 2005): 1553–1562.

Ref. 12:
Klunk, William E. MD, PhD, Henry Engler MD, Agneta Nordberg MD, PhD, Yanming Wang PhD, Gunnar Blomqvist PhD, Daniel P. Holt BS, Mats Bergström PhD, Irina Savitcheva MD, Guo-Feng Huang PhD, Sergio Estrada PhD, Birgitta Ausén MSCI, Manik L. Debnath MS, Julien Barletta BS, Julie C. Price PhD, Johan Sandell PhD, Brian J. Lopresti BS, Anders Wall PhD, Pernilla Koivisto PhD,

Gunnar Antoni PhD, Chester A. Mathis PhD, Bengt Långström PhD. "Imaging Brain Amyloid in Alzheimer's Disease with Pittsburgh Compound-B." *Annals of Neurology* 55, issue 3. (March 2004): 306–319.

Ref. 13:
Masliah E, Hansen L, Adame A, Crews L, Bard F, Lee C, Seubert P, Games D, Kirby L, Schenk D. "Abeta Vaccination Effects on Plaque Pathology in the Absence of Encephalitis in Alzheimer Disease." *Neurology* 64(1). (Jan 11, 2005): 129–31.

Ref. 14:
Patton RL, Kalback WM, Esh CL, Kokjohn TA, Van Vickle GD, Luehrs DC, Kuo YM, Lopez J, Brune D, Ferrer I, Masliah E, Newel AJ, Beach TG, Castaño EM, Roher AE. "Amyloid-Beta Peptide Remnants in AN-1792-Immunized Alzheimer's Disease Patients: a Biochemical Analysis." (September 2006).

Ref. 15:
Bruno Vellas, R. Black, Leon J. Thal, Nick C. Fox, M. Daniels, G. McLennan, C. Tompkins, C. Leibman, M. Pomfret, Michael Grundman. "Long-Term Follow-Up of Patients Immunized with AN1792: Reduced Functional Decline in Antibody Responders." Current Alzheimer Research 6 (2009): 144–151.

Ref. 16:
Gómez-Isla, Teresa, Joseph L. Price, Daniel W. McKeel Jr., John C. Morris, John H. Growdon, and Bradley T. Hyman. "Profound Loss of Layer II Entorhinal Cortex Neurons Occurs in Very Mild Alzheimer's Disease." *The Journal of Neuroscience* 16(14). (July 15, 1996): 4491–4500.

Ref. 17:
Kokjohn, Tyler A., Alex E. Roher. "Antibody Responses, Amyloid-β Peptide Remnants and Clinical Effects of AN-1792 Immunization in

Patients with AD in an Interrupted Trial." CNS Neurol Disord Drug Targets 8(2). (April 2009): 88–97.

Ref. 18:
Holmes C[1], Boche D, Wilkinson D, Yadegarfar G, Hopkins V, Bayer A, Jones RW, Bullock R, Love S, Neal JW, Zotova E, Nicoll JA. Lancet. "Long-term effects of Abeta42 Immunization in Alzheimer's Disease: Follow-Up of a Randomized, Placebo-Controlled Phase I Trial." 372(9634). (July 19, 2008): 216.

Ref. 19:
Louis Jacques, MD, Director, Coverage and Analysis Group, et al. Decision Memo for Beta Amyloid Positron Emission Tomography in Dementia and Neurodegenerative Disease (CAG-00431N). (September 27, 2013).

Ref. 20:
Golde TE1, Schneider LS, Koo EH. "Anti-aβ therapeutics in Alzheimer's disease: the need for a paradigm shift." *Neuron* 69(2). (Jan. 27, 2011): 203–13. doi: 0.1016/j.neuron.2011.01.002.

Ref. 21:
Sperling, Reisa A., et al. Toward defining the preclinical stages of Alzheimer's disease: Recommendations from the National Institute on Aging-Alzheimer's Association workgroups on diagnostic guidelines Table B2 for Alzheimer's disease. (May 7, 2011).

Ref. 22:
Hardy JA[1], Higgins GA. "Alzheimer's Disease: the Amyloid Cascade Hypothesis." *Science* 256(5054) (April 10, 1992):184–5.

Ref. 23:
Karran E, Mercken M, De Strooper B. "The Amyloid Cascade Hypothesis for Alzheimer's Disease: an Appraisal for the Development of Therapeutics." (August 2011).

Ref. 24:
Selkoe, Dennis J. "Resolving Controversies on the Path to Alzheimer's Therapeutics." *Nature Medicine* 17. (September 2011): 1060–1065. doi: 10.1038/nm.2460.

Ref. 25:
Sperling, Reisa A., M.D., Clifford R. Jack, Jr., M.D., and Paul S. Aisen, M.D. "Testing the Right Target and the Right Drug at the Right Stage." *Science Translational Medicine* 3(111) (Nov. 30, 2011). 111cm33.

Ref. 26:
Sperling, Reisa A., Dorene M. Rentz, Keith A. Johnson, Jason Karlawish, Michael Donohue, David P. Salmon, and Paul Aisen. "The A4 Study: Stopping AD before Symptoms Begin?" *Science Translational Medicine.* 6(228) (March 19, 2014): 228fs13.

Ref. 27:
Cummings, Jeffrey L., Travis Morstorf, and Kate Zhong. "Alzheimer's Disease Drug-Development Pipeline: Few Candidates, Frequent Failures." Alzheimer's Research & Therapy. 2014. doi: 10.1186/alzrt269.

Ref. 28:
Donohue, Michael C. PhD, Reisa A. Sperling, MD, David P. Salmon, PhD, Dorene M. Rentz, PsyD, Rema Raman, PhD, Ronald G. Thomas, PhD, Michael Weiner, MD, Paul S. Aisen, MD. "The Preclinical Alzheimer Cognitive Composite: Measuring Amyloid-Related Decline." *Original Investigation.* (August 2014).

Ref. 29:
De Strooper, Bart. "Lessons from a Failed γ-Secretase Alzheimer Trial." *Cell* 159, issue 4. (November 6, 2014): 721–726.

Ref. 30:
"Semagacestat Failure Analysis: Should γ-Secretase Remain a Target?" (Feb. 25, 2015).

Ref. 31:
"New Imaging Data Tells Story of Travelling Tau." Alzheimer's Association International Conference 2015. (Aug. 14, 2015).

Ref. 32:
Kandel, Eric, James H. Schwartz, Thomas M. Jessell, Steven A. Siegelbaun, A. J. Hudspeth. *Principles of Neural Science, Fifth Edition.* 2013.

Ref. 33:
Yang, Weili, Zhuchi Tu, Qiang Sun, and Xiao-Jiang Li. "CRISPR/Cas9: Implications for Modeling and Therapy of Neurodegenerative Diseases." *Frontiers in Molecular Neuroscience.* (April 28, 2016). doi: 10.3389/fnmol.2016.00030.

Ref. 34:
"Coming to a Center Near You: GAP and to Revamp Alzheimer's Trials." Alzheimer's Association International Conference 2016. (Aug. 11, 2016).

Ref. 35:
"Tau PET Studies Agree—Tangles Follow Amyloid, Precede Atrophy." Alzheimer's Association International Conference 2016. (Aug. 22, 2016).

Ref. 36:
Jack, Clifford R. Jr., Marilyn S. Albert, David S. Knopman, Guy M. McKhann, Reisa A. Sperling, Maria C. Carrillo, Bill Thies, Creighton H. Phelps. "Introduction to the Recommendations from the National Institute on Aging-Alzheimer's Association Workgroups on Diagnostic Guidelines for Alzheimer's Disease." *Alzheimer's & Dementia* 7 (2011): 257–262S.

Ref. 37:
"Tau PET Aligns Spread of Pathology with Alzheimer's." *Staging*. (March 11, 2016).

Ref. 38:
"Alzheimer's Disease and Related Dementias Research Implementation Milestone Database." NIH → National Institute of Aging.

Ref. 39:
Braak H[1], Braak E.Acta. "Neuropathological Staging of Alzheimer-Related Changes." *Neuropathology* 82(4). (1991): 239–59.

Ref. 40:
Ultsch, Mark, Bing Li, Till Maurer, Mary Mathieu, Oskar Adolfsson, Andreas Muhs, Andrea Pfeifer, Maria Pihlgren, Travis W. Bainbridge, Mike Reichelt, James A. Ernst, Charles Eigenbrot, Germaine Fuh, Jasvinder K. Atwal, Ryan J. Watts & Weiru Wang. "Structure of Crenezumab Complex with Aβ Shows Loss of β-Hairpin." *Nature*. (December 20, 2016).

Ref. 41:
"Alzheimer's in a Dish? Aβ Stokes Tau Pathology in Third Dimension." (Oct. 12, 2014).

Ref. 42:
"Genetic Wild West: 23andMe Raw Data Contains 75 Alzheimer's Mutations." (July 11, 2017).

Ref. 43:
"Test Finally, a Blood for Alzheimer's?" Alzheimer's Association International 2017 Conference. (July 28, 2017).

Ref. 44:
"Computational Modeling—Will it Rescue AD Clinical Trials?" (May 13, 2015).

Ref. 45:
"End of the EXPEDITION: Solanezumab Results Published." (Jan. 24, 2018).

Ref. 46:
Citron, Martin, Tilman Oltersdorf[†], Christian Haass, Lisa McConlogue, Albert Y. Hung, Peter Seubert, Carmen Vigo-Pelfrey, Ivan Lieberburg & Dennis J. Selkoe. "Mutation of the β-amyloid precursor protein in familial Alzheimer's disease increases β-protein production." *Nature* 360. (December 17, 1992): 672–674. doi: 10.1038/360672a.

Ref. 47:
Samson, Kurt. "Investigative PET Tracer for Tau Works in Living Alzheimer's Patients and Normal Adults." *Neurology Today*. (April 7, 2016).

Ref. 48:
"Dosage, A4 Researchers Raise Solanezumab Lengthen the Trial." (June 9, 2017).

Ref. 49:
Walsh, Dominic M., Dennis J. Selkoe. "Aβ Oligomers—a Decade of Discovery." (January 4, 2007).

Ref. 50:

Wang, Lixia, Fei Yi, et al. "CRISPR/Cas9-mediated targeted gene correction in amyotrophic lateral sclerosis patient iPSCs." (April 11, 2017).

Ref. 51:
"AD-Related Dementias Summit 2016: Progress, Aims, Dollars." Alzheimer's Disease-Related Dementias 2016 Summit. (April 20, 2016).

Ref. 52:
"Three's Company: Florbetaben Approved, Excludes AD Diagnosis." (May 02, 2014).

Ref. 53:
"Reaching for a Cure—ADRD Bypass Budget Proposal for FY 2017." NIH Bypass Budget Proposal for Fiscal Year 2017.

Ref. 54:
"Pittsburgh compound B History." (September 2007).

Ref. 55:
"Selecting Trial Participants Based on Tangle Pathology Might Improve Power." (March 18, 2017).

Ref. 56:
Karran, Eric, Marc Mercken and Bart De Strooper. "The amyloid cascade hypothesis for Alzheimer's disease: an appraisal for the development of therapeutics."

Ref. 57:
"CRISPR Gene Editing—Poised to Revolutionize Neuroscience?" Back to the Top (Sept. 12, 2014).

Ref. 58:
"Tau-PET in Down's: Unique Patterns Among Alzheimer's Types and Stages Clinical Trials on Alzheimer's Disease." (Dec. 22, 2016).

Ref. 59:
National Alzheimer's Project Act. Public Law 111-375. (Jan. 4, 2011).

Ref. 60:
"CRISPR Gene Editing—Poised to Revolutionize Neuroscience?" Back to the Top (Sept. 12, 2014).

Ref. 61:
"Stopping Alzheimer's Disease and Related Dementia." NIH Bypass Budget—Advancing Our Nation's Research Agenda Proposal for Fiscal Year 2018.

Ref. 62:
"Sustaining Momentum: NIH Takes Aim at Alzheimer's Disease & Related Dementias." NIH Bypass Budget Proposal for Fiscal Year 2019.

SECTION 3

Appendix

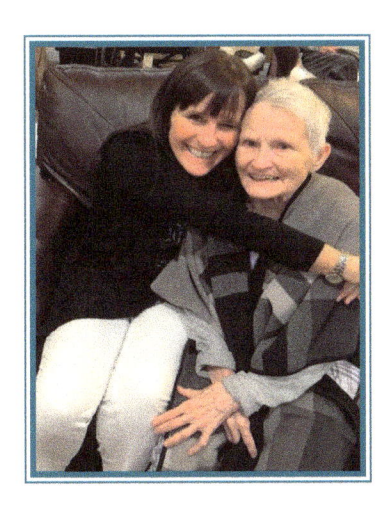

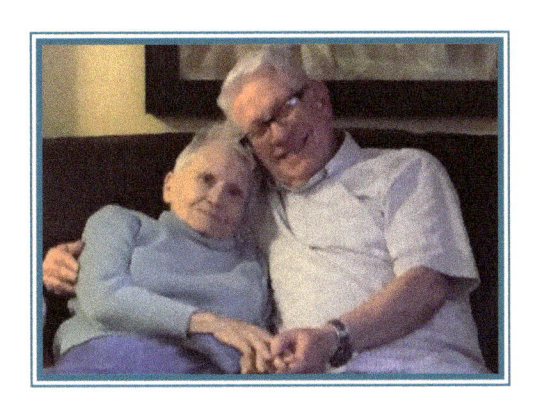

APPENDIX A

Definitions

Acetylcholine
An organic chemical that functions in the brain and body, as a neurotransmitter.

Acetylcholinesterase
An enzyme that breaks down unused acetylcholine in the synaptic cleft (the space between neurons). This enzyme is necessary to restore the synaptic cleft so it is ready to transmit the next nerve impulse.

Agitation
An emotional state of excitement or restlessness

Allele
Any one of a series of two or more different genes (from the mother and father) that occupy the same position on a chromosome). Autosomal chromosomes are paired (one from the egg and one from the sperm), each autosomal action is represented twice. If both chromosomes have the same allele, occupying the same location, the condition is referred to as homozygous for this allele.

If the alleles at the two locations are different, the individual or cell is referred to as heterozygous for both alleles.

Antigens

Substances which are capable, under appropriate conditions, of inducing a specific immune response and of reacting with the products of that response, that is, with specific antibodies or specifically sensitized T-lymphocytes, or both. Antigens may be soluble substances such as toxins and foreign proteins, or particulates such as bacteria and tissue cells.

Antioxidants

In biochemistry and medicine, antioxidants are enzymes or other organic substances such as vitamin E or beta-carotene, that are capable of counteracting the damaging effects of oxidation in tissue.

Anxiety

An emotion characterized by an unpleasant state of inner turmoil, often accompanied by nervous behavior such as pacing back and forth.

Apathy

A lack of feeling, emotion, interest, and concern

Aphasia

An inability to comprehend and formulate language, which can cause impairments in speech and language modalities. The four modalities are auditory comprehension; verbal expression; reading and writing; and functional communication.

ARMS

A group or subgroup of participants in a clinical trial that receives a specific intervention/treatment, or no intervention, according to trial protocol.

Astrocytes

The third class and most numerous neuroglial cells in the brain and spinal cord. Astrocytes (from "star" cells) are irregularly shaped with many long extensions including those with "end feet" which form the glial membrane and directly and indirectly contribute to the blood-brain barrier and the synapse activity where they regulate the extracellular ionic and chemical environment, and the immune system's "reactive astrocytes" (along with microglia) which respond to injury.

Autosomal Alzheimer's Disease

AD resulting from an inherited mutation in either the Amyloid Precursor Protein (APP) or the Presenilin 1 and 2 genes that causes an excess production of Beta Amyloid peptides.

Axon

A long projection of a neuron, that carries efferent (outgoing) action potentials from the cell body toward target cells. A nerve cell communicates with another nerve cell by transmitting signals from the branches at the end of its axon. At the terminal end of the axon, the impulses are transmitted to other nerve cells or to effector organs.

Beta Amyloid

A peptide of the Amyloid Precursor Protein consists of either 40, or 42 amino acids (AB_{40} or AB_{42}). AB_{40} is a soluble form. AB_{42} is a plaque form.

Blood-brain Barrier

A protective barrier formed by the blood vessels and glial cells of the brain. It prevents some substances in the blood from entering brain tissue.

Brainstem Hemorrhage

Hemorrhage in the Pons, often secondary to brainstem distortion due to rapidly expanding intra-brain lesions.

Catalyze
To speed up a chemical reaction.

Cell Division
The process by which a parent cell divides into two or more daughter cells.

Cerebrospinal Fluid
A clear, colorless fluid that contains small quantities of glucose and protein.
Cerebrospinal fluid fills the ventricles of the brain and the central canal of the spinal cord.

Cysteine
A semi-essential protein generated amino acid.

Delirium
A set of symptoms identified by a confused state such as attention deficits, disorganization of behavior, altered sleep-wake cycle, and/or psychotic features such as hallucinations and delusions.

Delusion
A belief held with strong conviction despite superior evidence to the contrary.

Depression
A state of low mood and aversion to activity.

Dimers
Dimers are two monomers. In proteins, dimers are two amino acids.

Disinhibition
In psychology, disinhibition is a lack of restraint manifested in disregard for social conventions, impulsivity, and poor risk assess-

ment. Disinhibition affects motor, instinctual, emotional, cognitive, and perceptual aspects.

Domain

Describes a part of a molecule or structure that shares common chemical features.

Dysphoria

Profound state of unease or dissatisfaction.

Endosome

A membrane-bound compartment inside a cell.

Enzyme

A protein molecule produced by living organisms that catalysis chemical reactions of other substances without itself being destroyed or altered upon completion of the reactions.

Etiology

Etiology is the study of causation or origination.

Euphoria

Pleasant excitement along with the sense of ease and well-being.

Essential Amino Acids

An amino acid that cannot be produced by the organism (brain), and thus must be supplied in a diet. The nine amino acids humans cannot produce are phenylalanine, valine, threonine, tryptophan, methionine, leucine, isoleucine, lysine, and histidine (i.e., F V T W M L I K H)

Free Radical

A chemically active atom or molecular fragment containing a chemical charge due to an excess or deficient number of electrons.

Genes
　Located in the nucleus of the cell, genes contain genetic information that is transferred from cell to cell.

Gene Product
　RNA or protein that results from the expression of a gene.

Glia
　Supportive tissue of the brain. There are three types of glial tissue: astrocytes, oligodendrocytes, and microglia. Glial cells do not conduct electrical impulses, as opposed to neurons.

Glial Cell
　Specialized cells that surround neurons, providing mechanical and physical support and electrical insulation between neurons.

Hallucination
　A perception in the absence of external stimulus that has qualities of a real perception.

Hyperphosphorylation
　Occurs when a biochemical with multiple phosphorylation sites is fully saturated and is one of the signaling mechanisms used by the cell to regulate mitosis.

Inflammation
　A localized protective response elicited by injury or destruction of tissues, which serves to destroy, dilute or wall off (sequester) both the injurious agent and the affected cells.

In vitro
　Parts of an organism within a glass, observable in a test tube, in an artificial environment.

In vivo

The effects of various biological entities, that are tested on whole, living organisms, usually animals, including humans, and plants.

Intervention

A process or action that is the focus of a clinical study. Interventions include drugs, medical devices, procedures, vaccines, and other products that are either investigational or already available. Interventions can also include noninvasive approaches such as education or modifying diets and exercise.

Lability (Psychological term)

Something that is constantly undergoing change or something that is likely to undergo change (e.g., emotional incontinence: a type of effect characterized by involuntary crying or uncontrollable episodes of crying).

Lipids

Biological molecules, soluble in nonpolar solvents, but only very slightly soluble in water. They are a heterogeneous group (being defined only on the basis of solubility) and include fats, waxes and terpenes.

Lymphocyte

A subtype of white blood cell in the immune system.

Luminal

The interior of a vessel such as the central space in an artery or vein.

Membrane

A selective barrier that allows some things to pass through but stops others.

(Think of a membrane as a traffic light functionally, and materially as Saran wrap.)

Metabolism
　　The set of life-sustaining chemical transformations within the cells of living organisms.

Microglia
　　Small glial cells which migrate through nerve tissue and remove waste products by phagocytosis.

Mitochondria
　　Small intracellular organelle which are responsible for energy production and cellular respiration.

Mitosis
　　Cell division of the nucleus.

Molecule
　　An electrically neutral group of two or more atoms held together by chemical bonds.

Monomer
　　Mono=one, mer=part—is one part that joins another part through a chemical reaction to form a molecule. (Protein Monomer is one amino acid. DNA Monomer is one nucleotide.

Neuroblastoma
　　Cells arising by division of precursor cells in neural ectoderm (formations during early brain development) that subsequently differentiate to become neurons.

Neurofibrillary Tangles
　　Aggregates of hyperphosphorylated tau protein.

Neurotransmitter
　　A chemical released by nerve cells to send signals to other cells.

Nucleotide

In DNA, it is an A, T, C, or G. (A=T and G=C). A is adenine; T is thymine; G is guanine; and C is cytosine.

Oligomer

(Oligo = few,—mer = parts) A polymer molecule composed of two, three and four monomers. In proteins, oligomers are a few dimers.

Oligomerize

Chemically join individual monomers into dimers and then into oligomers.

Oxidation

A chemical reaction in which oxygen combines with another element and the oxidation states of atoms are changed.

Parenchyma

The essential elements of an organ, used in anatomical nomenclature as a general term to designate the functional elements of an organ, as distinguished from its framework or stroma.

Peptide

A segment of a protein that consists of one to fifty amino acids.

Polypeptide

A segment of a protein that has more than fifty amino acids.

Phenotype

The observable physical or biochemical characteristics of an organism.

Phosphorylation

The addition of a phosphate to amino acids that causes a protein to become a target for binding or interacting with a distinct set of other proteins that recognize the phosphorylated domain.

Phosphorylation happens to many enzymes and structural proteins in the process of cell signaling.

Polypeptide

Polypeptide is a segment of a protein that has more than fifty amino acids.

Praxis

The process by which a theory, lesson, or skill is enacted, embodied, or realized.

Precursor

One that precedes and indicates the approach of another.
1. In biological processes, a substance from which another, usually more active or mature substance is formed.
2. In clinical medicine, a sign or symptom that heralds another.

Prodromal Alzheimer's Disease

A presymptomatic class of people who have been identified with amyloid in the brain through a PET scan.

Protease

Enzyme that begins catabolism by splitting of interior peptide bonds in a protein.

Proteins

The principal constituents of all cells are of high molecular weight and consist essentially of combinations of a long chain of amino acid peptide linkages.

Twenty different amino acids are commonly found in proteins and each protein has a unique, genetically defined amino acid sequence which determines its specific shape and function. They serve as enzymes, structural elements, hormones, immunoglobulins, etc.

Secretase

An enzyme that cleaves amyloid beta-precursor protein to generate three putative forms (alpha, beta, and gamma); beta and gamma enzymes form the beta amyloid peptide from the precursor, while alpha form cleaves the precursor so no beta-peptide forms.

Stroke

A condition due to the lack of oxygen to the brain which may lead to reversible or irreversible paralysis. The damage to a group of nerve cells in the brain is often due to interrupted blood flow, caused by a blood clot or blood vessel bursting. Depending on the area of the brain that is damaged, a stroke can cause coma, paralysis, speech problems, dementia, or death.

Synapse

Physiology: A connection between excitable cells, by which an excitation is conveyed from one to the other. Chemical synapse: one in which an action potential causes the transfer of neurotransmitter from the presynaptic cell, which navigates across the synaptic cleft and binds to ligand gated ion channels (a receptacle) on the post synaptic cell.

T-cell

A class of lymphocytes involved primarily in controlling cell-mediated immune reactions and in the control of B-cell development. The T-cells coordinate the immune system by secreting hormones.

Thymus

Lymphoid organ in which T lymphocytes are educated, mature and multiply.

Thymic hormone

Endocrinology: One of the hormones produced by the thymus that are believed to play a role in the maturation of T-lymphocytes and overall modulation of the immune system.

T-lymphocytes
Lymphoid cells concerned with cell-mediated immunity. They originate from lymphoid stem cells that migrate from the bone marrow to the thymus and differentiate under the influence of the thymic hormones.

Zymogen
An inactive precursor of an enzyme. Particularly, it is a proteolytic enzyme that breaks down a protein into polypeptides. Synthesized (produced) in the cell and secreted in this safe form, then converted to the active form.

APPENDIX B

Websites

ADAS-COG
https://www.verywell.com/alzheimers-disease-assessment-scale-98625

Alzforum
http://www.alzforum.org/

Alzheimer's Association
https://alz.org

Bruce Bauer's Web Site
alzheimersabcs.com

Center for Medicare and Medicaid Services
https://www.cms.gov/medicare-coverage-database/details/nca-decision-memo.aspx?NCAId=265

Disability Assessment for Dementia (DAD)
http://www.dementia-assessment.com.au/function/DAD_manual.pdf

The Dependence Scale for Alzheimer's Disease
http://www.todaysgeriatricmedicine.com/news/ex_112211_03.shtml

Healthy Brains
https://healthybrain.org

Lewy Body Dementia
http://www.nia.nih.gov/alzheimers/publication/lewy-body-dementia/common-symptoms

National Alzheimer's Project Act
https://www.congress.gov/111/plaws/publ375/PLAW-111publ375.pdf

National Institute of Aging—Bypass Budget Archive
https://www.nia.nih.gov/about/bypass-budget-proposal-archive

National Institute of Health (NIH)—Alzheimer's Disease
https://clinicaltrials.gov/search/term=alzheimer?JServSessionId-zone_ct=ktgk7i1tb1&Term=alzheimer&submit=Search

The PubMed government database website
https://www.ncbi.nlm.nih.gov/pubmed/

Teepa Snow
www.LBDtools.com

Wikipedia
https://en.wikipedia.org/wiki/Main_Page

APPENDIX C

Alzheimer's Disease (AD) Timeline

350 BC: Aristotle proposed that genetic material is carried in sperm.

1858: Charles Darwin's *On the Origin of Species* was published.

1866: George Mendel's pea experiment showed particulate nature of genetic determinants.

1869: Frederic Miescher discovered DNA.

1892: Senile plaques observed for the first time.

1895: Albrecht Kossel finds DNA is a long polymer of nucleotides A, T, G, and C.

1898: Austrian neurologist Emil Redlich related senile plaques with senile dementia.

1903: Chromosomes identified in dividing cells as the probable carriers of genes.

1906: Dr. Alois Alzheimer first described "a peculiar disease."

1910: Alzheimer's disease named by psychiatrist Emil Kraepelin, Dr. Alois Alzheimer's mentor.

1931: Invention of electron microscope allowed further study of brain.

1944: Oswald Avery experiment isolated DNA as a genetic material.

1953: James Watson and Francis Crick proposed the double helix structure of DNA.

1953: Alfred Hershey and Martha Chase performed tests proving DNA is genetic material.
1958: A carrot cloned from a single specialized cell.
1959: The roles of messenger RNA and transfer RNA in genetic expressions described.
1961: The first codon identified in the genetic code, relating the messengers in RNA to the amino acids in proteins.
1968: Measurement scales are developed for assessing cognitive and functional decline in older adults.
1974: The American National Institute on Aging (NIA) was established.
1975: Tau protein identified as heat stable protein, essential for microtubule assembly (axons and dendrites).
1980: The Alzheimer's Association began.
1982: Atomic Force Microscope (AFM) was invented by Gerd Binnig and Heinrich Rohrer, who received the 1986 Nobel Prize for physics.
1984: Beta Amyloid (AB_{42}) was identified as a peptide in amyloid plaque.
1984: Human Genome project was proposed.
1986: Tau protein was identified as a key component in neurofibrillary tangles.
1987: The amyloid precursor protein (APP) gene, from which beta-amyloid forms is identified on chromosome 21.
1989: The atomic force microscope (AFM) is commercially introduced.
1990: Start of the Human Genome Project (HGP) to determine sequence of nucleotide base pairs in human DNA.
1991: Braak's six stages of the entorhinal (EC) is published, including an autopsy report that indicated AD starts in the EC, and amyloid plaque starts 10 to 20 years before symptoms appear
1992: Presenilin-1 (PS-1) gene is identified.
1992: Alzheimer's "Amyloid Cascade Hypothesis" was published by John A. Hardy and Gerald A. Higgins.
1992: Familiar Alzheimer's disease (FAD) is identified as APP mutation that increases production of beta amyloid.

1993: ApoE gene on chromosome 19 is identified as the first gene that raises risk for Alzheimer's disease through its E4 allele.
1993: Presenilin-2 (PS-2) was discovered.
1993: FDA approves tacrine (Cognex), the first drug specifically targeting memory and thinking AD symptoms.
1995: First transgenic mouse model is developed for AD.
1996: Donepezil approved for use in all stages of AD.
1997: Discovered that tau mutation causes FTD (but not AD).
1998: Illumina Inc. is formed to provide integrated systems, to analyze DNA sequencing in the lab.
1999: AN-1792 AB antibody: immunotherapy for AD in a mouse model; clears plaques.
2001: Galantamine approved for mild to moderate stages of AD.
2002: Terminated phase two immunotherapy AB vaccine trial due to brain inflammation in 6% of patients.
2003: Memantine approved for moderate to severe stages of AD.
2003: Stated completion of the Human Genome Project.
2004: Pittsburgh Compound B (PIB), a radioisotope imaging agent that can be detected by positron emission tomography (PET), provided a breakthrough in disease monitoring and early detection.
2004: AD Neuroimaging Initiative (ADNI) began a nationwide study to establish standards for obtaining and interpreting brain images.
2011: New criteria and guidelines for Alzheimer's disease diagnosis, and a proposed research agenda to define a new preclinical stage are proposed.
2012: Dominantly Inherited Alzheimer Network (DIAN) begins a clinical trial to prevent the onset of AD in people who inherited an autosomal dominant high risk mutation.
2012: CRISPR/Cas9 is discovered as a tool to modify gene DNA mutations.
2012: AMYVID is approved as an amyloid radioisotope imaging agent for PET scans.
2013: Bapineuzumab lowers brain Aβ load in AD patients but misses primary endpoints in phase 2 while lowering CSF tau.

2013: VIZAMYL becomes the second amyloid radioisotope, imaging agent approved for PET scans.
2014: Alzheimer's in a Dish model created in the laboratory of Rudolph Tanzi.
2017: A blood biomarker to measure brain amyloid was reported by Dr. Randall Bateman.

APPENDIX D

AN-1792 Case Study

AN-1792 Concept

This 2001 Phase two-a clinical trial used a synthetic beta amyloid peptide (AB42) to activate the brain's immune system to clear out amyloid plaques from the brain through normal brain functions.

NIH Trial #NCT00021723

Structure

A two-year trial designed for 375 patients started in September 2001. Twenty-seven study sites were in the USA and Europe, which included sites in the UK, Switzerland, Spain, and France.

Goals

1. For volunteers who received the vaccine, their immune system would produce antibodies to attack the amyloid plaque and remove it from the brain.

2. Patient cognitive functions would improve.
3. Patient' symptomatic behavior would improve.
4. Safety would be demonstrated.

Goal Result
1. Patients developed antibodies. Some
2. Plaque cleared from the brain. Failed
3. Improved cognitive functioning. Debatable
4. Improved symptomatic behavior. For two patients
5. Safety demonstrated. Failed

Date—Event

January 23, 2002: Four patients have fallen ill with what appears to be central nervous system inflammation. (Ref. 3)

February 25, 2002: *The Washington Post* reported last Friday (January 22, 2002) that a dozen more patients in the suspended trial of the Aβ Vaccine AN-1792 have now fallen ill with cerebral inflammation. (Ref. 4)

Post-Trial Analysis

Both AN-1792 phase one and phase two-a trials factor into this case study. Research analysis and reports offered a debatable source of data. Bruce has selected following segments to discuss and provide his views of the reported analysis by researchers. The segments are AN-1792 phase one, AN-1792 phase two-a, trial termination, meningoencephalitis, AN-1792 phase two-a meningoencephalitis, AN-1792 Phase two-a autopsy, AN-1792 phase two-a one-year follow-up, AN-1792 phase two-a long-term follow-up, AN-1792 vaccine trials open issues, Bruce's comments and AN-1792 summary.

AN-1792 Phase One

AN-1792 phase 1 was a safety and tolerability trial of eighty volunteers with mild and moderate Alzheimer's disease (AD). The results showed the vaccine was well-tolerated, and tests indicated that some patients developed amyloid antibodies. A follow-up trial from September 2003 to September 2006 confirmed evidence that the AN-1792 vaccine initiated a neuro-immune response that disrupted amyloid plaque. (Ref. 18) The phase 1 follow-up provided evidence that amyloid disruption had no effect on stopping or delaying neurodegeneration. From September 2001 to September 2006, forty-two of the eighty participants died. Autopsies of seven of eight patients, who showed virtually complete plaque removal, had severe end stage dementia before death. (Ref. 18)

AN-1792 Phase 2-a Trial

A multicenter, double-blind, placebo-controlled out-patient, safety, tolerability and pilot efficacy study. (NIH ID $: NCT00021723)

The study enrolled 370 volunteers with mild to moderate Alzheimer's disease at investigational sites in the United States and Europe. Volunteers received either AN-1792 or a placebo, and they were evaluated using standard clinical assessments of cognition and memory as well as experimental surrogate markers of AD pathology. The goal of the study was to evaluate the clinical impact of eliciting an immune response (formation of antibodies) to the synthetic Abeta peptide in volunteers with AD. The trial started in September 2001 with an estimated completion of September 2003. However, the trial was suspended temporarily on January 23, 2002, because four patients had fallen ill with what appeared to be central nervous system inflammation. (Ref. 3) A safety committee terminated the trial at the end of February 2002 after an additional twelve patients developed meningoencephalitis. (Ref. 4)

Trial Termination

After the trial terminated at the end of February 2002, meningoencephalitis was found in eighteen of the 300 patients vaccinated. [Refs. 11] Of the three hundred vaccinated patients, only fifty-nine responded with their immune system generated antibodies. Therefore, 80 percent of the vaccinated patients had no immune system response to the synthetic Abeta peptide vaccine. Post-trial reporting focused on the fifty-nine (20 percent) who responded, and primarily on the eighteen (33 percent) of the fifty-nine responders with meningoencephalitis. A woman with meningoencephalitis in the UK died ten months later.

Since the failed AN-1792 vaccine trial was such a major event, there were many outstanding analysis reports by the research community. Opinions varied from challenging support for the amyloid cascade hypothesis to support for continuing its pursuit. There was even one voice for presymptomatic candidates [Ref. 6], which never was a consideration in 2003. It took another decade to be accepted.

Meningoencephalitis

When the AN-1792 trial terminated, eighteen volunteers had been diagnosed with meningoencephalitis. What is that?

Meningoencephalitis is a combination of meninges and encephalitis. Encephalitis is an acute inflammation of the brain. Meninges are three layers of membranes that function between the skull and the neurons in the brain. The meninges area contains body cells as opposed to neurons, and functions under the body's immune system as opposed to the brain's immune system. Therefore, T-cells and macrophages perform the functions like microglia do in the neural system.

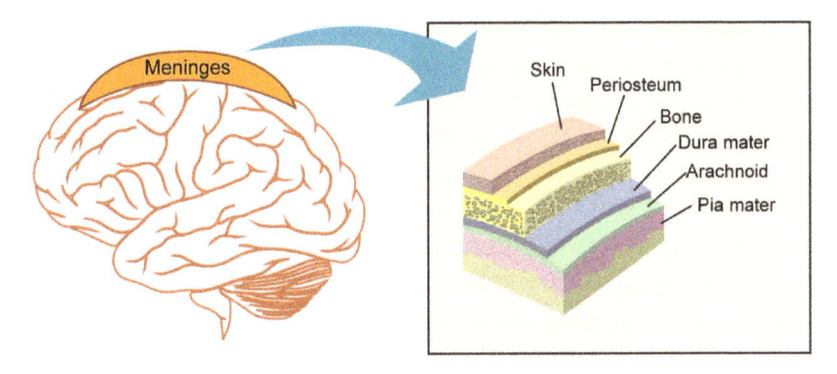

Fig. D.1. Meninges.

The meninges consist of three layers: the dura mater, the arachnoid mater, and the pia mater. The primary function of the meninges and of cerebrospinal fluid is to protect the central nervous system. The combination of the Arachnoid and the Pia is the leptomeninges. This was the area where encephalitis occurred in the eighteen patients during the AN-1792 trial.

The dura mater is a thick, durable membrane closest to the skull. It contains larger blood vessels that split into the capillaries in the pia mater. The middle element of the meninges is the arachnoid mater. This thin, transparent membrane is composed of fibrous tissue and, like the pia mater, is thought to be impermeable to fluid. The pia mater is a very delicate membrane that firmly adheres to the surface of the brain and spinal cord.

To explain AN-1792 termination, along with the impact of the result, it is necessary to separate a *neuro-immune response* from a *plasma (blood vessels) immune response*. AN-1792 phase 2-a meningoencephalitis will cover the plasma (blood) immune response. The neuro-immune response and the many debatable issues then follow.

AN-1792 Phase 2-a Meningoencephalitis

This adverse event terminated the trial, but also illustrated the complexity of finding an intervention. (Ref. 3, Ref. 14, Ref. 17)

Meningoencephalitis occurred in eighteen patients. The cause of the inflammation was not determined. Whether the AN-1792 vaccine caused the activation of the plasma-immune response to attack amyloid plaque in blood vessel (cerebral amyloid angiopathy—CAA) and/or release T-cells and macrophages (blood cells equivalent to microglia in the neuro-immune system) in response to inflammation is uncertain. Beta amyloid can incite inflammatory neuro-immune responses, but whether this type of inflammation promotes, or counterbalances neurological damage is unclear. (Ref. 7)

Whether the plasma system reacted to a neuronal-caused inflammation, or whether the plasma system caused the inflammation, has not been determined. In any event, eighteen patients experienced the inflammation condition—meningoencephalitis. Evidence of both neuro-immune response (microglia) as well as a plasma-immune response (T-cells) complicated analysis. (Ref. 7) Sixteen of the eighteen patients had received two doses, one had received one dose, and one had received three doses of the study drug before symptoms occurred. The median latency from the first and last injections to symptoms was seventy-five and forty days. (Ref. 7) Twelve patients recovered to, or close to, baseline within weeks, whereas six remained with disabling cognitive or neurologic sequelae (continuing decline symptoms). (Ref. 7)

AN-1792 Phase 2-a Autopsy

The UK segment reported on an autopsy performed on the patient who died from the meningoencephalitis after ten months. (Ref. 5) She had committed her brain for autopsy. The autopsy evidence was the following: (a) There were extensive areas of neocortex with very few Abeta plaques. (b) Those areas of cortex that were devoid of Abeta plaques contained densities of tangles, neuropil threads, and cerebral amyloid angiopathy (CAA) similar to unimmunized AD but lacked plaque-associated dystrophic neurites and astrocyte clusters. (c) In some regions devoid of plaques, Abeta-immunoreactivity was associated with microglia. (d) T-lymphocyte meningoencephalitis was present. And (e) cerebral white matter showed infiltration by macrophages. Findings (a-c) strongly resemble the changes seen after Abeta immunotherapy in mouse models of AD and suggest that the neuro-immune response generated against the peptide-elicited clearance of Abeta plaques in this volunteer. (Ref. 5)

Bruce's Comments: It appears that the neuro immune system responded and dissolved plaque and produced antibody tithers. It seems the body immune system responded and breeched the brain/blood barrier (BBB). There were no postulates of why the body's immune system breeched the BBB and produced T-cells, macrophages. Does this inconclusive report of a significant adverse event (SAE) illustrate the need for increase knowledge relative the brain's immune system and its interaction with the body's immune system?

Biochemical Analysis of Amyloid-Beta Peptide Remnants (Ref 14):

Neuropathological examination of volunteers vaccinated against purified Aβ42 (AN-1792) demonstrated that senile plaque disruption occurred in immunized humans. Tissue was examined under the microscope and then quantified. It biochemically characterized the remnant amyloid peptides in the gray and white matter and leptomeningeal/cortical vessels of two AN-1792-vaccinated volunteers, one of whom developed meningoencephalitis. Compact core and diffuse amyloid deposits in both vaccinated individuals were focally absent in some regions (plaque dissolved).

Although parenchymal (*brain as opposed to vascular/arteries*) amyloid was focally disaggregated, vascular deposits were relatively preserved or even increased. Immunoassay revealed that total soluble amyloid levels were sharply elevated (*from the dissolved plaque*) in vaccinated patient gray and white matter compared with Alzheimer's disease cases. (Earlier reports didn't reveal this.)

These experiments suggest that although immunization disrupted amyloid deposits, vascular capture (*veins absorbed the soluble amyloid*) prevented large-scale egress (*removal*) of Abeta peptides. Trapped, solubilized amyloid peptides may have had a cascading toxic effect on cerebrovascular, gray, and white matter tissues.

Anti-amyloid immunization may be most effective not as therapeutic or mitigating measures but as a prophylactic (*preventative*) measure when Abeta deposition is still minimal (*MCI and Pre-Symptomatic*). This may allow Abeta mobilization under conditions in which drainage and degradation of these toxic peptides is efficient.

AN-1792 Phase 2-a One Year Follow-Up

One year after termination, Swiss researchers conducted their own assessment of 28 of their original 30 cohorts (two dropped out). (Ref. 8) Elan decided to keep the terminated Phase II-a trial at a blind status, until they could conduct a follow-up trial. (Ref. 18)

A one-year follow-up assessment in the AN-1792 Phase II-a study by Swiss researchers reported in May 2003 that volunteers who were antibody responders showed improvements in one-year cognitive measures as assessed by a nine-component neuropsychological test battery (NTB—a composite of tests assessing memory and executive function). (Ref. 8) Of the twenty-eight volunteers, nine with little or no antibodies were considered the control group (volunteer data was still blinded). Three of the other nineteen were responders developed meningoencephalitis. Of those nineteen responders, thirteen received an intermediate dose and six received a strong dose. Whereas control volunteers worsened, the intermediate group only declined slightly, and the strong group remained stable. These data establish the possibility that antibodies against β-amyloid were effective in halting the progression of AD. (Ref. 8) Two volunteers had improved MMSE scores of 28 and 30, from 25 and 24 at baseline, respectively.

Considering today's (2017) emphasis toward presymptomatic intervention, Bruce considers this improvement to have been an overlooked early messenger.

Responders demonstrated significantly less impairment in "activities of daily living tests" and significantly less dependence on caregivers compared with the control patients. (Ref. 4, Ref. 8)

Sid Gilman of the University of Michigan, Ann Arbor, offered a different view, saying that, "Overall, they did not find significant differences between the placebo and responder groups from baseline versus 12 months." (Ref. 6) However, NTB tests did show favorable responders results in the visual section. These were independent site reports without having the data unblinded by Elan.

AN-1792 Long Term Follow-Up

After approximately 4.6 years, a multi-centered follow-up, out-patient study, was conducted from January to October 2006. Two hundred fifty-one original volunteers participated. Changes in volunteer living situation since the beginning of the phase 2-a study and any serious adverse events (SAEs) that occurred after the last visit in the initial phase 2-a study, were determined. Functional tests were by telephone with caregiver and capable volunteers. Volumetric brain MRI results revealed a decrease in whole brain volume (WBV) and an increase in ventricular volume in antibody responders compared with placebo-treated volunteers. (Ref. 15) Shrinkage in cortex and hippocampus coupled with enlargement of the ventricles implies that AD is getting worse (Ref. 9).

The following functional and cognitive assessments were performed: Disability Assessment for Dementia (DAD), Dependence Scale, Clinical Dementia Rating—Sum of Boxes (CDR-SOB), MMSE, NTB, and Alzheimer's Disease Assessment Scale Cognitive Subscale (ADAS-Cog.

Functional Results

DAD

Caregivers provided DAD ratings for 27 of the 30 placebo-treated v0lunteers (90.0 percent) and twenty-four of the twenty-five antibody responders. After approximately 4.6 years of follow-up, antibody responders demonstrated a 25.0 percent lower decline in activities of daily living as determined by the DAD compared with placebo-treated patients. (Ref. 15)

Dependence Scale

Caregivers provided Dependence Scale ratings for twenty-eight of the thirty placebo-treated volunteers (93.3 percent) and twenty-four of the twenty-five antibody responders (96.0 percent). Antibody responders demonstrated a 17.6 percent lower mean score in caregiver dependence compared with placebo-treated patients. (Ref. 15)

CDR-SOB

Clinical Dementia SOB ratings were obtained for 24 of the 30 placebo-treated volunteers (80.0 percent) and twenty-two of the twenty-five antibody responders (88.0 percent). Like the DAD and Dependence Scale, antibody responders showed 20.2% less decline on the CDR-SOB scale compared with placebo, although this difference was not statistically significant. (Ref. 15)

COGNITIVE RESULTS

NTB (Neuropsychological Test Battery)

At the time of the follow-up study, the NTB was attainable in only ten of the thirty placebo-treated volunteers (33.3 percent) and thirteen of the twenty-five antibody responders (52.0 percent). No significant differences were observed in the change, from baseline, for the overall NTB 9-component z score between antibody responders and placebo-treated volunteers. (Ref. 15)

Mini-Mental State Examination (MMSE)

MMSE was attainable in eighteen of the thirty placebo-treated volunteers (60.0 percent) and twenty of the twenty-five antibody responders (80.0 percent). No significant differences were observed between antibody responders compared with placebo-treated patients after 4.6 years of follow up. (Ref. 15)

ADAS-Cog

ADAS-Cog was attainable in eleven of the thirty placebo-treated volunteers (36.7 percent) and sixteen/twenty-five antibody responders (64.0 percent). No significant differences in ADAS-Cog scores were observed between placebo-treated patients and antibody responders after approximately 4.6 years of follow up. (Ref. 15)

In contrast to testing of functional and cognitive measures, (for which caregiver assessments were available for most participating subjects) fewer assessments of cognitive outcomes (including the NTB, MMSE, and ADAS-Cog) were able to be performed as volunteers became less amenable to, or were unable to undergo, cognitive evaluation due to disease progression. (Ref. 15) Furthermore, antibody responders' cerebrospinal fluid (CSF) tau levels showed a reduction, compared with placebo-treated volunteers, which suggested a reduced level of neurodegeneration. (Ref. 15)

AN-1792 Vaccine Trials Open Issues

1. AN-1792 inflammatory response: Whether this inflammation promoted or counterbalanced neurological damage was unclear. (Ref. 6)
2. What was the meaning of CSF Tau decrease? In the small subset of phase 2-a subjects who had CSF examinations, CSF tau decreased in antibody responder vs placebo subjects. (Ref 11) An autopsy showed the antibodies did not clear the damage of tau neurofibrillary tangle that already existed. Cognitive symptoms correlate with tau neurofibrillary tan-

gles internal to cell nuclei, which were unaffected. (Ref. 6) What caused decrease in CSF tau and what did it mean?
3. Atrophy of responder's brain remains an unexplained issue.
4. The missing link issue: Loss of tau correlates with cognitive symptoms. Amyloid does not correlate with cognitive symptoms. The link between amyloid and tau is still elusive.

Bruce's Comments

The results of data analysis appear to have been "in the eye of the beholder." Some claims of benefits. (Ref. 5, Ref. 8, Ref. 15) *Some claim of no benefits.* (Ref. 11) *The termination of the trial by an adverse event was unfortunate for research but very significant to those who developed meningoencephalitis.*

1. *Were mild and moderate patients too far demented to benefit from amyloid intervention? The entorhinal cortex (EC) plays a crucial role as a gateway connecting the neocortex and the hippocampal formation. The EC is affected severely in Alzheimer's disease, likely initiating memory impairment. There are (±) 7 million neurons in the adult human EC. No significant loss of neurons in the EC is detectable in cognitively normal subjects between the sixth and ninth decades of life. By contrast, a very severe neuronal loss (estimated 32 percent) in the EC is found in very mild AD cases. These are at the threshold for clinical detection of dementia. This neuronal loss is so marked that it must have started well before onset of clinical symptoms. The degree of neuronal loss in the EC parallels incidences of NFTs and neuritic plaques, but not diffuse plaques without neuritic changes. The results highlight the need to develop new diagnostic tests to predict the pre-symptomatic and very mild stages of AD before massive neuronal loss in select neural populations has occurred, when therapeutic intervention might be most effective.* (Ref. 16) *Does this 1995 data suggest patients are*

too demented for effective intervention when symptoms first appear?

2. *Two apparent trial design insufficiencies were never recognized or accepted as such. By targeting efficacy toward improvement and/or cure, the design criteria accepted only volunteers with mild or moderate AD. As published in reference 10, these volunteers were too far demented for expected intervention success. Unfortunately, tools were not yet available to pursue presymptomatic candidates. Also, though a link was confirmed between amyloid and tauopathy, evidence for the amyloid cascade causing hyper-phosphorylation of tau and neuron death was (and continues to be) elusive. Did the design criteria of accepting mild and moderate volunteers contribute to the next decade of failed trials? The second insufficiency was the questionable effectiveness of cognitive measuring tools. Again, unfortunately, the tools used were insufficient, although the best available. Consider how many neurons are lost when a volunteer reaches a moderate stage of AD. Like a stroke victim, to regain lost neurons, new pathways must be connected. That takes time and the learning function, which also may no longer be available at the moderate stage. Do volunteers in the moderate stage of the disease have too much neuron damage to demonstrate any improvement? The questions, in the cognitive tools used in the AN-1792 were effective for broad decline changes rather than incremental change needed for efficacy. Elicited answers from volunteers or caregivers became too judgmental to determine small changes. Reviewers of the data also introduced uncertainties. Computer models being used for data analysis today were not available.*

3. *Results from the AN-1792 phase 1 follow-up trial provided an "outside the box" indicator—reported but never emphasized or recognized. Two patients with MMSE scores of 25 and 24, and whose immune systems generated antibodies, showed improvement, with new MMSE scores of 30 and 28 respectively. Could this be the type of improvement or delay expected in pre-symptomatic patients if plaque is dissolved or prevented*

from aggregation? Were the patients early enough in the disease decline process that damage was not too far advanced? (Ref. 8) *Was this a missed opportunity not to have followed these two? How long would the anti-bodies remain effective (if they ever were) before neurodegeneration reappeared, if ever?*

4. *The quality of the functional test data in the phase 2-a 4.6-year follow-up is questionable. Most patients were apparently in the severe stage of AD during the January to October 2006 follow-up and unable to participate in the testing. Therefore, most of the responses were caregiver subjective inputs.* (Ref. 15) *Could the claim of functional improvement also be somewhat subjective?*

5. *The AN-1792 phase 2-a cognitive results indicated no significant difference between responders and placebo volunteers. This was not surprising with the MMSE scores in the 8–12 range (Severe stage). At this range, volunteers have lost all memory, executive functions of thinking, comprehension, and learning. As wonderful a tool the MMSE is for broad decline, it is not a tool for detecting small incremental change over weeks, months, or even years, depending on disease stage such as mild cognitive impairment or very early mild AD.*

6. *Phase 2-a patients were incapable of cognitive testing, which raises questions as to the neurodegenerative benefits claimed in the one-year follow-up study. Was the claim of cognitive benefits in Phase I made questionable by the adjustment to the control group from six placebos to a group of nine that included selected responders? Could the overall Phase I data be questionable?*

7. The phase 2-a functional test inputs were mostly by caregivers, thus being subjective. Lacking was data comparing individual volunteers by MMSE scores. This would have allowed assessing the degree of decline by MMSE scores for each volunteer in the mild and moderate groups. Then, comparison could have indicated whether early stage patients (MMSE 26) benefited as responders compared to moderate patients (MMSE 15). Such results might have

shown the need to change trial design criteria away from moderate volunteers. Does degree of decline play a role in measuring the volunteer's capability to benefit from vaccine or any drug? Do MMSE scores of 15 or 17 or 19 indicate decline has gone too far for any efficacy? The failed trials of the past decade seem to indicate such results, along with a design criteria strategy switch to candidates who have pre-symptomatic conditions, mild cognitive impairment (MCI), or mild AD.

AN-1792 Summary

The AN-1792 clinical trials provided scientifically beneficial results of knowledge regarding amyloid plaque. Numerous published reports debated many of the results found. Significant optimism was reported in early preliminary reports that were debated in final analysis.

Benefits

1. The benefits were "in the eye of the beholder."
2. Proponents of the amyloid cascade hypothesis (ACH) saw results as supportive and rational for continuing ACH pursuit.
3. The possible real benefits were lost by the myopic pursuit of ACH. (See Bruce's Comments.)

Evidence

1. AN-1792 vaccine activated a neuro-immune response that disrupted/dissolved amyloid plaque of volunteers with mild and moderate AD. (Ref. 13)

2. The disruption of amyloid plaque did not prevent or delay the progressive neurodegeneration of AD.
3. AN-1792 vaccine causes whole brain shrinkage in antibody responders.
4. AN-1792 vaccine had no significant effect on cognitive functions.
5. Abeta immunotherapy-associated reduction was confined to neuronal processes. (i.e., neuropil threads and dystrophic neurite). (Ref. 10)
6. P-tau accumulation in the neuronal cell bodies (nucleus), contributing to neurofibrillary tangles, appeared not to be affected. (Ref. 10)

Quote of the Trial

Dr. Roger M. Nitsch, Professor, Faculty of Medicine, University of Zurich, Switzerland said, *"It was a shock to us, who believe it takes 10 years for a plaque to develop, to see it disappear within three days after a single dose of antibody,"*

APPENDIX E

PET Scan Tracers

PET Scan Tracers Approved by the FDA

Tracer name		Type of Target	ApprovedDate	RadioIsotope	Developer
Technical	Commercial				
Florbetapir	Amyvid	Amyloid	July 2012	Fluorine-18(F-18)	Avid Radio-pharmaceuticals
Flutemetamol	Vizamyl	Amyloid	October 2013	F-18	GE Healthcare
Florbetaben	Neuraceq	Amyloid	March 2014	F-18	Piramal (Ref. 52)

PET Scan Tracers Under Development

Tracer Name		Type of Target	Status	RadioIsotope	Developer
Technical	Commercial				
T807, Flortaucipir	AV1451	TAU		F-18	Eli Lilly/Avid
Fluselenamyl		Amyloid		F-18	Wash U. ST. L
Ro695894811C]		TAU	Phase 1		F. Hoffman- La Roche (Ref. 31)
RO6924963		TAU			
11C]RO6931643		TAU			
MK-6240		TAU			MERCK
PI-2620	MNI-960	TAU			Piramal Imaging
	Jnj-067	TAU			JANSEN

About the Author

Bruce Bauer is an eighty-five-year old retired engineer, caregiver, silver-smith, and jewelry maker who has been married to his wife Ethel for fifty-seven years through which they have two children and five grandchildren.

Bruce grew up in St. Louis, Missouri, and served his country during the Korean War. Upon his honorable discharge, he used the GI Bill of Rights to graduate in three and a half years with a bachelor of science in electrical engineering from the Missouri School of Mines and Metallurgy, in January 1959.

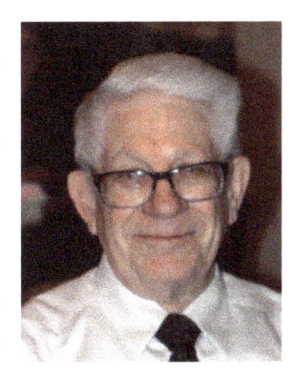

Bruce spent a thirty-two-year career with General Electric in engineering and engineering management. Assignment included flight testing a bombing computer on the F-105 aircraft, design and management of checkout equipment for the Instrument Unit on the Apollo Launch Vehicle. He concluded his professional career in management of nuclear energy research.

Bruce carried his work ethics and desires for learning and increasing his knowledge into retirement. He developed a habit of exercising to where today, after over twenty-five years, he still exercises twelve hours per week.

Retirement learning came in many ways, beginning with traveling the world. Using new lapidary skills to convert many semi-precious rocks, he added gold and silver-smiting to his skill set to make jewelry. This was followed by making stain glass windows for his home and friends, producing paternal and maternal genealogy documents for family members, and, finally, his self-education of Alzheimer's disease and dementia.

Bruce's past seventeen years of learning not only included a self-education on Alzheimer's disease but writing monthly articles on the disease and the Brain, teaching a class on Alzheimer's and dementia, and addressing the Alzheimer's Foundation of America 2017 Conference in Las Vegas, NV, as a caregiver.

As this book is being published, Bruce is developing a web site, whereby he can continue to provide his views on AD and Alzheimer's Disease Related Dementia (ADRD) to the public.